Nurses' Aids Series
SPECIAL INTEREST TEXT

CARDIAC NURSING

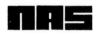

NURSES' AIDS SERIES

SPECIAL INTEREST TEXTS

Nurses' Aids Series
SPECIAL INTEREST TEXT

Cardiac
Nursing

David R. Thompson, SRN, ONC, RMN

Charge Nurse, Coronary Care Unit,
The General Hospital, Leicester

with a foreword by
PAT ASHWORTH, MSc, SRN, SCM, FRCN
Research Programme Manager,
WHO Collaborating Centre,
Department of Nursing,
University of Manchester

BAILLIÈRE TINDALL · LONDON

Published by BAILLIÈRE TINDALL,
a division of Cassell Ltd,
Greycoat House, 10, Greycoat Place, London SW1P 1SB

an affiliate of
Macmillan Publishing Co. Inc.
New York

First published 1982

ISBN 0 7020 0900 8

Typeset by Academic Typesetting, Gerrards Cross, Bucks
Printed in Great Britain by Nene Litho
Bound by Woolnough Bookbinding Ltd.,
Wellingborough, Northants.

British Library Cataloguing in Publication Data

Thompson, David R.
   Cardiac nursing.——(Nurses' aids series, Special
   interest text)
   1. Cardiovascular disease nursing
   I. Title   II. Series
   616.1'2'0024613   RC674
ISBN 0-7020-0900-8

Contents

FOR MY FATHER

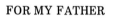

Foreword

Nursing has been affected in the last thirty to forty years by a number of changes in medical science and technology, and in society and the people who need nursing care. This is particularly so in relation to heart disease. It is one of the major causes of death and disability among relatively young adults as well as the increasing number of elderly people in western society, yet an increasing amount is becoming known about how to prevent or treat it, and nurses have a major contribution to make to this.

Developments in medical knowledge and technology have presented nurses with the challenge to learn to use these within the context of nursing care, without allowing technical functions to displace care of the whole person. It is also beginning to be recognized that nurses, wherever they work, should be helping people to remain or become more healthy as well as caring for the sick; by teaching and assisting them to maintain healthy life-styles and avoid known hazards as well as cope with disability when necessary.

To assess the need for such care, and to plan, implement and evaluate it, nurses require a good basis of knowledge in addition to their basic desire to care for people and technical and interpersonal skills. David Thompson has gathered together a range of such knowledge and combined it with his experience of cardiac patient care to provide a very useful guide and reference source. It now remains for those who read it to apply this in developing increasingly good nursing practice, for nurses should be developing nursing deliberately rather than just responding to outside pressures.

Finally, to my good wishes for the success of this book I would add the hope that those reading it will find as much joy and satisfaction in cardiac nursing as the author and many others of us have done.

April, 1982   PAT ASHWORTH

Preface

In writing this book I have attempted to produce an account of modern cardiac nursing which is complete enough to be coherent, but simple enough to be comprehensive to those with little knowledge of cardiology. I have concentrated on providing up-to-date information in sufficient detail to meet the needs of most nurses and for a list of common cardiocascular abbreviations used in the text the reader is referred to page 278. Although a book of this size cannot hope to encompass all aspects of modern cardiac nursing, it is hoped that it will stimulate the interest of nurses to go deeper into the subject.

Congenital heart disease is an entity of its own and, therefore, only very brief mention is made of it within the confines of this book. The Nursing Process approach to patient care has been used, but it has to be appreciated that only the fundamental aspects are mentioned. For a much more detailed account the reader is referred to one of the many excellent texts available.

April, 1982   DAVID R. THOMPSON

Acknowledgements

I am greatly indebted to my friend Professor Robert Anderson, Cardio-thoracic Institute, University of London, for his constant encouragement and great enthusiasm shown in this work. Without his help this book would never have materialized.

I am grateful to Dr James Fleming for his comments on some of the medical aspects, and I must thank my friends and colleagues, in particular Mr G.S. Bowman, Nursing Officer, for their constant interest and advice on the nursing aspects. Also the staff of the Department of Medical Illustration, Leicester Royal Infirmary for all their help.

Thanks are also extended to my publishers, Baillière Tindall, particularly to Rosemary Long, Nursing Editor, for her patience and help.

Finally, I must thank those dear to me who suffered many silent and irritable hours.

Kind permission has been given to reproduce figures as follows: Figs 21, 23, 34–46, 48 and 60, Cambridge Instruments Ltd.; Fig. 53, Cardiac Recorders Ltd.; Fig. 59, Paladin Medical Products Ltd.; Figs 51 and 55, Dr Michael Sumerling, Consultant Radiologist, Freeman Hospital, Newcastle-upon-Tyne.

DAVID R. THOMPSON

1
Historical Introduction

The heart has always held a special place in man's estimation and has been the subject for scientific writers since Egyptian, Greek and Roman times. One of the reasons why the anatomy and physiology of the heart took so long to develop was the lack of satisfactory metaphors for thinking about what was seen. The written evidence of early Greek science is so fragmentary that it gives an unreliable picture of what was known or believed.

Aristotle made important embryological investigations and asserted that the first signs of life in a hen's egg are noticeable on the third day, the heart being visible as a pulsating sac. He considered the heart the first organ to live and the last to die. He placed the seat of intelligence in the heart and refused to attach any great importance to the brain. He also stated that the heart could not contract any disease.

Galen laid the foundations of a biological attitude to the heart. However, he thought that the blood freely traversed the heart, and failed to take into account the septum. Vesalius later demonstrated this, but because of traditional theory insisted that the blood 'sweated' across the septum through pores. The most significant contradiction to Galen's theories were the principles of blood flow in the veins, especially valvular function, later demonstrated by Harvey in his famous experiment.

Leonardo disproved Galen's theory of the pulmonary vein conveying air to the heart, and later proved that the valves in the heart allowed the blood to pass in one direction only.

Servetus, the Spanish philosopher–theologian suggested that the blood made its way from the right side to the left through a 'northwest passage' in the lungs. Columbus was more exact and stated that the blood was carried to the lung via the pulmonary artery.

William Harvey was the first modern biological scientist. He reconsidered some of the other traditional assumptions of the actions of the heart. Traditional theories demonstrated the misunderstanding of the mechanics of muscular contraction. Harvey's dissertation on the movement of the heart and blood is one of the greatest scientific texts. In it, Harvey laid the foundation of the sciences of experimental physiology and experimental medicine. (*De Motu Cordis, 1628*)

The capillary vessels were first demonstrated in 1661 by Malpighi using the microscope. By now the attitudes of Galen and Aristotle towards the heart and great vessels had passed into the shadow.

Diseases of the heart were not recognized until post-mortem examinations were permitted by the Church in the sixteenth century. Cardiology as such did not exist until well into the twentieth century. However, a considerable number of physicians made particular observations in the physiology and diseases of the heart and blood vessels. The most notable included the description of the oxygenation of the blood by Mayow in 1668; the identification of intra-cardiac post-mortem clots by Kerckring in 1670; pulmonary oedema due to mitral stenosis by Vieussens in 1715, and right ventricular hypertrophy and failure by Lancisi in 1728. Descriptions of the use of quinine in the control of cardiac arrhythmias, and of that of opium and venesection in cardiovascular emergencies were made by Senac in 1749.

A detailed description of angina pectoris was made by Herberden (1768), and digitalis was introduced for heart failure by Withering (1785). A detailed study of the nerves of the heart was carried out by Scarpa (1794). The invention of the stethoscope by Laennec (1819) revolutionized the diagnosis of heart disease. A description of chronic constrictive pericarditis was made by Chevers (1844); the first human electrocardiogram was performed by Waller (1877); and a description of a small bundle of conducting tissue in the fibrous ring was made by His (1893). Roentgen (1895) had invented the X-ray radiograph — the first one of the heart occurred in the late 1890s. Mackenzie (1902) invented an ink-polygraph to correlate pulses in arteries and veins with the heart beat. Einthoven (1903) invented the string galvanometer thus allowing the introduction of clinical electrocardiography. Keith and Flack (1907) discovered what they believed to be the heart's pacemaker, a fact verified by Lewis (1910), who later carried out important physiological and clinical studies with the electrocardiogram (1920).

By now, advances in medicine were being rapidly achieved. Souttar (1923) had attempted to open the mitral valve; Hyman (1932) had developed the first effective cardiac pacemaker, and the discovery of anticoagulants came about two years later. Gross (1938) surgically corrected a persistent ductus arteriosus, and surgery of the major peripheral blood vessels, and great vessels of the heart became frequent in the 1940s. Cournand (1941) and Richards (1945) were studying patients with the technique of cardiac catheterization, following its development by Forssmann (1929). Fleming (1946) had discovered penicillin — which was purified and adapted for therapeutic use by Florey and Chain in 1941. Blalock and Taussig (1945) had devised a surgical technique for the palliation of congenital malformations of the heart. Hufnagel (1954) developed the first artificial heart valve, and successfully inserted it in the descending aorta (Rose et al 1954).

Cardiac surgery really began in the 1950s when the heart/lung machine (Gibbon 1954) was perfected and became more reliable. Heart transplantation became a modern possibility mainly due to the work on animal heart transplants done by Guthrie and Carrel (1907). Lower and Shumway (1960) published their findings of perfecting a method of removing the heart in experiments in dogs. In 1964, Hardy et al transplanted the heart of a chimpanzee into man; an act unduly criticised at the time. Barnard (1967) shocked the world with the first successful human allograft, closely followed by a second. Six months later, Ross (1968) performed Britain's first heart transplant. In 1969, bio-engineers produced an artificial heart composed of plastic and dacron which was later implanted by Cooley et al (1969).

Meanwhile, other significant advances had been made. Although Vesalius (1543) had written about cardiac resuscitation in the sixteenth century, it was Igelsrud (1901) who successfully resuscitated an arrested heart. Beck et al (1947) reported successful defibrillation using electric current, and Kouwenhouven et al (1960) reported successful closed chest cardiac massage. The introduction of beta-adrenergic blocking drugs (Dornhorst and Robinson 1962; Black et al 1964) was a major advance. The concept of intensive coronary care came into being in the early 1960s (Day 1963; Brown et al 1963; Julian et al 1964;

Meltzer 1964; Robinson et al 1964), followed by the introduction of mobile coronary care units (Pantridge and Geddes 1966). The upsurge of recognizing cardiac arrhythmias was remarkable, leading to the development of a vast range of cardiovascular drugs including anti-arrhythmic, vaso-dilator and anti-hypertensive agents. Radio-isotope and ultrasound diagnostic techniques soon followed. Hounsfield (1972) invented the whole body scanner, developed by EMI, and known as the CAT (Computerized Axial Tomography) scanner.

Rapid advances are occurring in medicine, perhaps more so in the field of Cardiology. Perhaps the most significant advance is that of the emphasis being placed on the prevention of heart disease.

IMPLICATIONS FOR THE NURSE

It would be useful for the nurse to know the important landmarks in history, as this would give her a greater insight into the field of cardiology. However, she should also realise that parallel to the changes in cardiovascular medicine, have been the changes that have occurred in the field of coronary care nursing. Change that is effective usually takes time, and is still occurring throughout the nursing profession. Nursing needs to continually redefine its functions in terms of patient needs rather than merely the sphere of traditional nursing.

HISTORICAL BACKGROUND

It was not until the era of Florence Nightingale (1820–1910) that nursing began to have structure and foundations, although it was still not regarded as a profession. From the Nightingale era to World War II scientific development in medicine was slow and the function of the nurse was clear and required little development by way of changing the role or function of the nurse. In post-war years scientific knowledge within medicine and medical technology greatly increased. During this period the nurse occupied her time trying to keep abreast of how this new knowledge was to be put into practice and spent much of her time supporting the aims and aspirations of her medical colleagues. In doing so, the behaviour and response of the nurse became stereo-typed and unthinking. It is only recently that the nurse has had the opportunity to consider and re-think her role with the result that she is at present agitating for change. These changes relate to the unique-ness of the nursing function and the autonomy the nurse should have over her own behaviour and response to the sick person. Developments of patient allocation, the nursing process, and in some areas the re-defining of the sister/charge nurse role, are part of the belief many nurses have in their usefulness to the patient.

An insight into the history of our professional development should give the nurse the desire to continue the development of her unique function through research and professional literacy so that she under-stands human behaviour, changes in society and medicine, thus evolving rational approaches to new problems.

THE IMPACT OF CORONARY CARE

The concept of coronary care had the greatest impact upon the nurse involved in cardiac nursing. The introduction of these specialized units brought about many changes in the role of the nurse. They were required to take on the additional responsibilities of ECG recording and interpretation, initiation of appropriate treatment, cardiopulmonary resuscitation and the general support given to the critically ill. These responsibilities required a great deal of knowledge and skill, and most nurses were inadequate in these. To help meet these educational and practical needs of the nurse, a new body, the Joint Board of Clinical Nursing Studies (JBCNS), was set up in 1970. This body organized post-registration courses, and decided the requirements of the hospital and organized the syllabus. The coronary care course (JBCNS course No. 124) has helped in meeting the needs of the nurse working in this area.

Until recently medical staff were delegating responsibilities to the nursing staff, who automatically assumed them. Demands on the nurses were high, and many of these units were becoming highly technical and impersonal. It is only recently that the nursing profession has re-examined its role. The nurse has become more aware of the patients psychological as well as physical needs and feels more competent in delivering health care. She now plays a unique role in preventive measures in heart disease, cardiac rehabilitation, and health education. The role of the nurse has expanded and encompasses all these aspects.

She now functions in the community as well as in the hospital. Nurses now play important roles in running counselling and rehabilita-tion clinics, health education, and exercise programmes.

REFERENCES

Barnard, C.N. (1967) The operation: A human cardiac transplantation. An interim report of a successful operation performed at Groote Schuur Hospital, Cape Town. *S. Afr. med. J.*, *41*, 271.

Beck, C.S., Pritchard, W.H. & Feil, H. (1947) Ventricular fibrillation of prolonged duration abolished by electric shock. *J. Am. med. Ass.*, *135*, 985.

Chain, E.B. (1954) The development of bacterial Chemotherapy. *Antibiotics & Chemotherapy*, *4*, 215.

Cournand, A.F. & Ranges, H.S. (1941) Catheterization of the right auricle in man. *Proceedings of the Society for Experimental Biology & Medicine*, *46*, 462.

Day, H.W. (1963) Preliminary studies of an acute coronary care area. *Lancet, ii*, 53.

Einthoven, W. (1903) Die galvanometrische Registrierung des menschlichen Elecktrokardiogramme: Zugleich eine Beurteilung der Anwendung des Capillar-electrometers in der Physiologie. *Pfugers Archiv. fur die gesamte Physiologie des Menschen und der Tiere*, *99*, 472.

Fleming, A. (1946) *History and development of penicillin.* In: *Penicillin: its practical application* (Ed. A. Fleming). Philadelphia: Blakiston Co.

Florey, H.W. (1946) The use of micro-organisms for therapeutic purposes. *Yale Journal of Biology & Medicine*, *19*, 101.

Gibbon, J.H. (1954) Application of mechanical heart & lung apparatus to cardiac surgery. *Minnesota Medicine*, *37*, 171.

Kouwenhoven, W.B., Jude, J.R., & Knickerbocker, G.G. (1960) Closed chest cardiac massage. *J. Am. med. Ass.*, *173*, 1064.

Lewis, T. (1920) *The mechanism and graphic registration of the heart beat.* London: Shaw and Sons.

Mackenzie, J. (1902) *The study of the pulse and movements of the heart.* London: Macmillan Publishers Ltd.

Partridge, J.F. & Geddes, J.S. (1967) A mobile intensive-care unit in the management of myocardial infarction. *Lancet, ii*, 271.

2
The Heart

NORMAL DEVELOPMENT OF THE HEART

During the first two months of embryonic life the cardiovascular system undergoes a series of changes, at the end of which it has largely assumed its adult pattern. (*Thompson and Anderson 1982b*)

Before the third week of development the embryo is so minute that it can receive nutrition by simple diffusion, and the entire development of the heart and great vessels occurs between the third and eighth week of fetal life. During the first two weeks of this period (i.e. the third to fifth week of fetal life), the heart develops from a single straight cardiac tube, which becomes twisted into an S-shape, and divides into five dilatations by constrictions in the tube. The dilatations are:

Sinus Venosus (into which the veins of the body drain)
Atrium
Ventricle
Bulbus Cordis (Conus Arteriosus)
Truncus Arteriosus

Later in development, *septa* appear which divide the atrial and ventricular chambers into the left and right parts. The septum between the two ventricles is complete, but that between the two atria is traversed by the *foramen ovale*. The atria and ventricles are separated by the ingrowth of tissue from the atrioventricular sulcus. The liberation of the subendocardial layer of the ventricles forms the mitral and tricuspid valves, which are attached to the annulus formed from sulcus tissue. A septum is formed in the bulbus cordis and the truncus arteriosus, dividing them into the outflow tracts of the ventricles and into the aorta and pulmonary artery.(*Anderson and Becker 1980*)

The heart of the human embryo is thought to begin beating about the twenty-third day after conception. In more readily studied embryo of animals, it has been observed that the first heartbeats are irregular and weak and that the embryonic blood supply moves in and out of both ends of the heart with each beat. Gradually the activity of the heart tube becomes more regular and forceful, and blood begins to flow in one direction through it, entering at the caudal end and leaving at the cranial end.

FETAL CIRCULATION

It is clear that the fetal circulation of blood differs significantly from circulation after birth.

The lungs are functionless during fetal life, and the blood supply to them is therefore minimal. The fetus obtains its nutrition across the placenta in which the maternal circulation runs close to the fetal circulation. The blood of the fetus becomes oxygenated in this way. It leaves the placenta by way of the *umbilical veins* which lead into the *ductus venosus*, a large vessel on the postero-inferior surface of the fetal liver. The ductus venosus then runs into the inferior vena cava and thus brings the arterial blood to the right atrium. Only a small fraction of the blood entering the right atrium reaches the right ventricle; most of it is deflected by the *eustachian valve* of the inferior vena cava, towards the atrial septum and through the foramen ovale to the left atrium, left ventricle and aorta. The venous blood returning to the right atrium via the superior vena cava, flows through the tricuspid valve into the right ventricle and thence into the pulmonary artery. However, because the fetus is not breathing, the lungs do not require much blood. Thus the blood is shunted from the pulmonary artery through the *ductus arteriosus* to the descending aorta. This becomes a channel for the venous blood leaving the fetus. It runs into the *umbilical arteries* which arise from the internal iliac arteries of the fetus, and these take the blood back to the placenta, where it is oxygenated once again.

At birth aeration and expansion of the lungs occur. Also, more blood flows back from the lungs to the left atrium, so the flap-like valve of the foramen ovale closes and seals up within a week. The midwife ties the umbilical cord, and the ductus arteriosus closes.

The physiological changes in the ductus arteriosus, ductus venosus, foramen ovale and umbilical vessels occur very rapidly, but the anatomical changes are more gradual. Several months elapse before the channels are completely obliterated, though the adult pattern of circulation is rapidly attained after birth. (*Shinebourne and Anderson 1980*)

ANATOMY OF THE HEART

GENERAL DESCRIPTION OF THE HEART AND PERICARDIUM

The heart is a hollow, muscular organ enclosed in a fibroserous sac, the *pericardium*. It is approximately conical in shape so that the *base* faces upwards, backwards and to the right, and the pointed *apex* points downwards, forwards and to the left. Due to this obliquity about two-thirds of the heart lies to the left, and one third to the right of the median plane. Its longitudinal axis forms an angle of about 45° with both the sagittal and horizontal planes.

The heart is placed behind the sternum and the adjacent parts of the

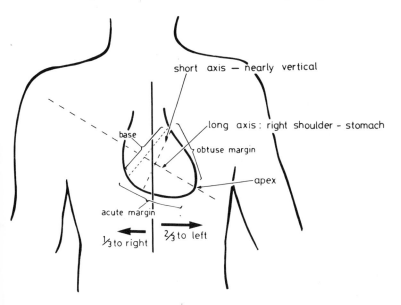

Fig. 1. *Diagram showing the position of the heart within the chest.*

costal cartilages in that part of the thorax known as the middle media-stinum. The pleural sacs with their contained lungs form the lateral relation of the heart on each side. The base is related to the vertebral column, oesophagus and descending aorta. The great vessels enter and leave at the base.

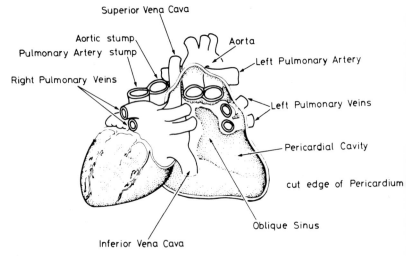

Fig. 2. *Position of the oblique sinus of the pericardium.*

Its size is closely correlated to the body size and corresponds quite accurately with the size of the clenched fist of the subject.

The heart has an *apex* and four surfaces, a *base*, a *sternocostal*, a *left* and a *diaphragmatic* surface. The borders of the heart are *upper*, *lower*, *right* and *left*. The sternocostal surface is separated from the diaphragmatic surface by the sharp lower border, and from the left surface by the rounded left border. The left border is formed almost entirely by the left ventricle, but at its upper part the left auricle enters into its formation. The right border is formed by the right atrium and the upper border, lying behind the commencement of the aorta and pulmonary trunk, by both atria but particularly the left. The base, formed mainly by the left atrium, is situated posteriorly opposite the 5th - 8th thoracic vertebrae. Of the four chambers of the heart, the two atria are mainly postero-superior, while the two ventricles are antero-inferior. The sternocostal surface facing upwards, forwards and to the left, is formed mainly by the right ventricle, with the addition of part of the right atrium and right auricle to its right, and a strip of the

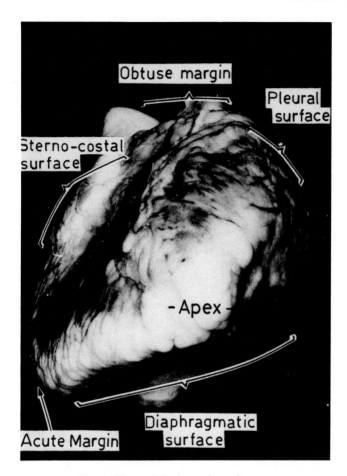

Fig. 3. *View of the heart from its apex.*

left ventricle to its left. The apex, situated at the junction of the left and lower border, is formed by the left ventricle and is at the level of the 5th left intercostal space, 9 cm from the mid-line. The diaphragmatic surface, resting mainly on the central tendon of the diaphragm, is formed mainly by the left ventricle. It fits into the cardiac notch of the left lung from which it is separated by the pericardium, pleura and phrenic nerve.

At about one-third of the distance from the base to the apex a *deep oblique groove* surrounds the heart and separates the atria from the

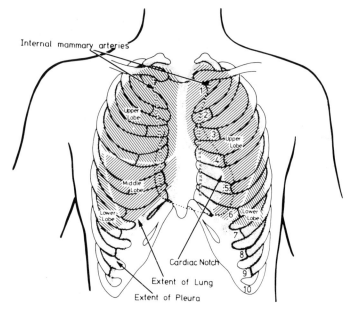

Fig. 4. *Relationship of the heart to the lungs and the internal mammary arteries.*

ventricles, the *atrioventricular groove* or *sulcus.* From the atrioventricular groove, two grooves extend towards the apex, one anteriorly — the *anterior interventricular groove*, and one posteriorly — the *posterior interventricular groove.* These mark the position of the ventricular septum and separate the right from left ventricles. The junction of the posterior interventricular and posterior atrioventricular grooves is known as the *crux.*

The heart is enclosed in a sac, the *fibrous pericardium* which serves to limit its sudden distension. Within the fibrous pericardium and on the surface of the heart, there is a thinner and more delicate membrane, the *serous pericardium.* This is divided into an outer or *parietal layer* which lines the inner surface of the fibrous pericardium, and an inner *visceral layer* or *epicardium*, which covers the outer surface of the heart and the adjoining portions of the great vessels. Where the great vessels pass through the fibrous pericardium, the two layers of the serous pericardium becomes continuous with one another, enclosing between them the pericardial cavity. In health the cavity contains only a small amount of fluid formed by the serous pericardium. There is just sufficient fluid to form a thin film on the smooth surface of both layers of

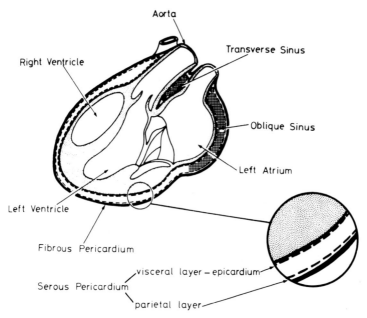

Fig. 5. *Structure of the pericardial cavity.*

the serous pericardium, thus acting as a lubricant to facilitate movements of the heart within the pericardial cavity.

The relations and attachments of the mediastinal structures to one another, as well as to the thoracic wall, have an important effect upon the position and movements of the heart. The fibrous pericardium blends with the tunica adventitia of the great vessels passing through it (aorta, pulmonary trunk, superior vena cava, inferior vena cava and pulmonary veins). It is also firmly attached to the central tendon of the diaphragm below and to the back of the sternum by the sterno-pericardial ligaments.

VARIATIONS IN SHAPE AND POSITION OF THE HEART

During life, the size, shape and position of the heart in the adult are subject to considerable variation. The heart tends to vary with the general physique of the individual and is influenced by its own physiological activity, as well as by movement of related structures, e.g. the diaphragm during respiration.

The shape of the chest and the level of the diaphragm usually vary with the body build. In the tall, thin type of individual (*asthenic* or *leptosomatic*) the chest is elongated and narrow and the heart is frequently described as *long*. In the short, stout type (*hypersthenic* or *pyknic*) the chest is short and wide and the heart is transverse. In the average individual (*athletic* or *asthenic*) the heart is characteristically *oblique*.

The position of the heart may be influenced by gravity, and the pressure of a distended stomach.

At birth the average heart weight is 20 – 25 g. The average weight of the normal adult heart is 280 – 340 g in the male, and 230 – 280 g in the female. The capacities of both ventricles are approximately the same, 90 – 120 ml. The atria are slightly less capacious.

The infant's heart is transverse in type, and appears to be very large in proportion to the transverse diameter of the chest. The heart is about 0.2% of the body weight, whereas in the adult it is about 0.43%.

After birth, the heart gradually changes in shape and relative size, and by puberty has attained its adult proportion.

INTERIOR OF THE HEART

Right atrium

This chamber has a relatively thin wall. It receives the superior vena cava, inferior vena cava, coronary sinus, venae cordis minimae and the anterior cardiac veins. The interior of the right atrium is smooth except on the anterior part of its wall and in the auricle, where transversely running ridges of the *musculi pectinati* appear. Posteriorly they end on a longitudinal elevation which runs from the right side of the orifice of the superior vena cava to the right side of the orifice of the inferior vena cava, called the *crista terminalis*. Entering the posterior portion of the right atrium are the *superior vena cava* above, and the *inferior vena cava* and *coronary sinus* below. The lower lateral margins of the inferior vena cava are guarded by the *eustachian valve*. The opening of the superior vena cava is not guarded by a valve. A smaller *coronary valve*, or *Thebesian* valve, guards the opening of the coronary sinus. The *right atrioventricular orifice* has a valve which possesses three cusps, hence the name *tricuspid valve*.

Scattered over the walls are the orifices of the *venae coridis minimae*, two or three small vessels, the *anterior cardiac veins* also open into the right atrium. On the interatrial septum there is a depression, the *fossa ovalis*. This fossa is the site of the foramen ovale of the fetus. It is not

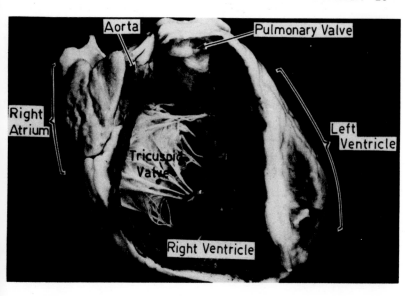

Fig. 6. *Heart dissected. View from the front showing position of the right-sided chambers.*

uncommon for a valvular opening between the two atria to persist throughout life.

Left atrium

This chamber is irregularly cuboidal in shape, somewhat smaller than the right atrium, and its walls is a little thicker. It receives the four *pulmonary veins* arranged in pairs each side, all four orifices devoid of valves. As in the right atrium, there are the orifices of the *venae cordis minimae*. The *left atrioventricular orifice* has a valve which possesses two cusps arranged like a bishop's mitre, hence the name *mitral valve*.

The interior of the left atrium is smooth, except in the auricle where the ridges of the *musculi pectinati* occur. There is no crista terminalis in this atrium. The left atrial aspect of the septum is roughened, being the flap valve of the fossa ovalis.

Atrioventricular junction

There is no muscular continuity between the atria and ventricles except through the conduction tissue of the atrioventricular node and bundle. The aortic and mitral valves have a strong, *fibrous ring*, continuous with a dense fibrous and fibrocartilaginous mass placed more deeply,

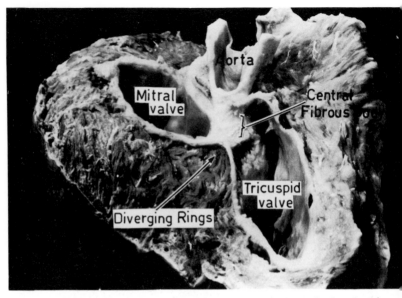

Fig. 7. *Oblique view of the fibrous skeleton from behind, showing the central body.*

sometimes called the *heart skeleton*. The pulmonary valve does not have a ring, and that of the tricuspid valve is only partially formed. These rings prevent the orifices from stretching and the valves from being rendered incompetent.

Right ventricle

This crescent-shaped chamber which normally expels blood against very low resistance has a relatively thin outer wall, but thicker than those of the atria. It is approximately one-third the thickness of the left ventricle.

This chamber forms the greater part of the sternocostal surface of the heart and its lower border, but the smaller part of the diaphragmatic surface. It communicates posteriorly with the right atrium through the *right atrioventricular orifice*, while anteriorly and above this is the *pulmonary trunk*. The left or septal wall bulges into its interior. The *pulmonary orifice* is guarded by the *pulmonary valve* which has three semi-lunar cusps named anterior, right and left. There are corresponding sinuses. The right atrioventricular, or tricuspid orifice is guarded by the *tricuspid valve* which has three flat triangular cusps, septal, anterior and inferior. Small accessory cusps are frequently present in the angles between these three cusps, and likewise consist of a fold of endocardium strengthened by fibrous tissue. The atrial surfaces, over which the entering blood flows, are smooth whereas the ventricular surfaces are roughened to give insertion to the chordae tendineae. The cone-shaped summit of the base of the right ventricle from which the pulmonary trunk arises is called the *infundibulum* or *conus arteriosus.* Blood entering the infundibulum is ejected superiorly and posteriorly into the pulmonary artery. The pulmonary valve is separated from the tricuspid valve by the *crista supraventricularis.*

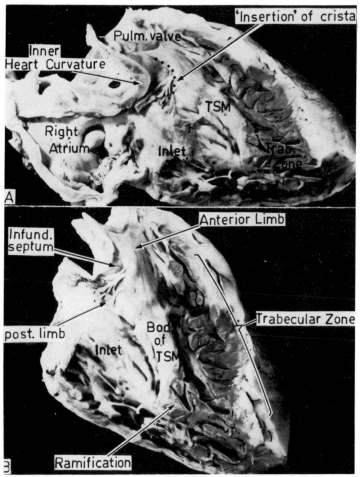

Fig. 8. *The right ventricular surface of the septum.*

On the inner surface of the ventricular wall are a number of irregular projections, the *trabeculae carneae*, formed by raised bundles of muscle fibres. Other muscle bundles, the *papillary muscles* project into the ventricular cavity to become continuous with the *chordae tendineae*, which are attached chiefly to the free border of the cusps of the tricuspid valve, and to a lesser extent, to their ventricular surface. Contraction of the ventricle not only apposes the cusps of the tricuspid valve, but also prevents their inversion into the atrium through the pull on the chordae tendineae.

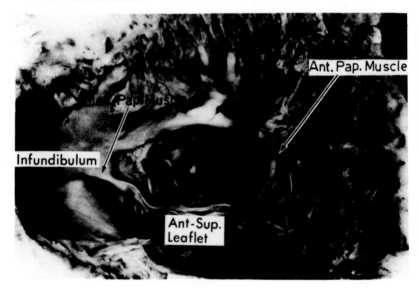

Fig. 9. *The infundibulum of the right ventricle.*

A large rounded muscle bundle, the *moderator band*, crosses the cavity of the right ventricle from the interventricular septum to the anterior wall.

Left ventricle

This chamber is conical, and its apex forms the apex of the heart. It normally expels blood against a much higher resistance than the right ventricle, therefore the wall of the left ventricle is approximately three times as thick as the right. During embryonic life, the ductus arteriosus is patent, and the walls of the right and left ventricles are more equal in thickness, but the left ventricle is still thicker.

Above and anteriorly, the left ventricle opens into the aorta. Below and posteriorly, it communicates with the left atrium through the *left atrioventricular orifice*. The right or septal wall is concave towards the cavity. The left atrioventricular orifice is guarded by the *mitral valve*, a bicuspid valve which has two triangular unequal cusps, anterior and posterior. The anterior cusp lies between the atrioventricular and aortic orifices and is frequently referred to as the aortic cusp of the mitral valve. The two *papillary muscles*, anterior and posterior, are much larger than those of the right ventricle. From these, *chordae tendineae* proceed to both cusps of the mitral valve.

In the posterior part of the *aortic vestibule*, which is the portion of the ventricular chamber immediately adjoining the commencement of the aorta, the aortic valve is in fibrous continuity with the mitral valve, there being no supraventricular crest. The *aortic orifice* is guarded by the *aortic valve* which has three semi-lunar cusps, right, left and posterior. They are stronger than those of the pulmonary valve. The wall of the aorta at the site of each cusp shows a slight dilatation or *sinus*. The right coronary artery arises from the *right aortic sinus*, and the left coronary artery from the *left aortic sinus*.

The orifice of each artery is above the level of the cusp. These three aortic sinuses are known as the *sinuses of Valsalva*.

The interventricular septum is thick and muscular for the most part, except for a small part, where it is thin membrane, the *membranous part of the septum*. This not only intervenes between the two ventricles, but to a slight extent its upper portion separates the right atrium from the left ventricle.

The *trabeculae carneae* are more numerous than in the right ventricle.

Valves of the heart

The main valves of the heart are the *mitral, tricuspid, aortic* and *pulmonary*. The arrangements have already been described. Valves are complex structures and are very strong, for example, during a normal lifetime they will open and close some 2700 million times. They have no blood vessels in health except perhaps at the bases of the atrioventricular valves.

TISSUES OF THE HEART

The main mass of the heart consists of muscular tissue or *myocardium*, lined by *endocardium* and covered by the visceral layer of serous pericardium or *epicardium*. There are blood and lymphatic vessels, nerves, varying amounts of fat and areolar tissue, and specialized conducting tissue.

Epicardium

This consists of a single layer of flat or low cuboidal mesothelial cells on a thin layer of loose connective tissue containing elastic fibres, small blood vessels and nerves. It is separated from the myocardium in places by a layer of adipose tissue which carries the coronary blood vessels of the heart.

Myocardium

Individual cardiac muscle cells are grouped in bundles in a connective tissue framework which carries small blood and lymphatic vessels and autonomic nerve fibres. The number of capillaries for each group of muscle cells is much greater than in skeletal muscle.

The myocardium in the atria and ventricles consists of a network of muscle fibres which show transverse and longitudinal striation, and which branch so as to connect with each other and act as a pseudosynctium. Once contraction starts in any part, it cannot remain localized but spreads throughout the entire network of muscle cells. There is a much greater amount of muscle in the ventricular walls than the atria, therefore the arrangement of fibres is more complex. The differences in ventricular thickness, results in the left ventricle having in effect a largely separate deep layer of muscle.

Endocardium

This is continuous with the lining of the vessels. It is much thinner than the epicardium and consists of a lining of endothelial cells, a middle layer of dense connective tissue containing many fine elastic fibres, and an outer layer of loose connective tissue in which there are small blood vessels and the specialized conducting tissue. The heart valves are also formed by folds of endocardium, thickened by a core of fibrous tissue extending in from the sulcus tissue.

CONDUCTING SYSTEM OF THE HEART

In addition to the purely contractile muscle fibres composing the atria and ventricles, the heart possesses certain 'specialized' tissues which form the conducting system. The initiation and conduction of impulses

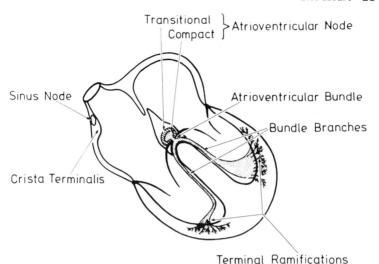

Fig. 10. *Diagrammatic representation of the conducting system of the heart.*

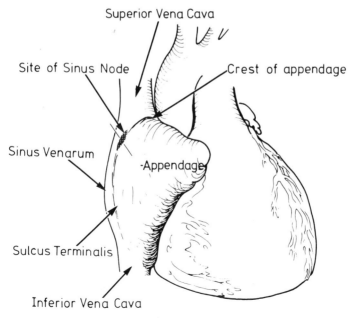

Fig. 11. *Diagram illustrating the position of the sinus node.*

for the contraction of the heart occurs with the specialized muscle cells
of this system. The conducting system consists of the following:

Sinus (S–A) node
Atrioventricular (A–V) node } *Atrioventricular*
Atrioventricular (A–V) bundle } *junction*
Right and left bundle branches } *Ventricular*
Peripheral ramifications of the bundle branches } *conducting tissue*

The human heart does not contain 'purkinje' cells. (*Thompson and Anderson 1982a*)

SINUS (S-A) NODE

The sinus node is the normal site of initiation of the inherent regular
rhythm. It is situated at the junction of the superior vena cava with the
right atrium (see Fig. 11). This junction appears on the epicardial surface as the sulcus terminalis, and on the endocardial surface as the
crista terminalis. The node is spindle-shaped, about 25 mm in length
and about 3 mm in width. It is fairly clearly demarcated.

The framework of the node is collagenous, interlaced by bundles of
fibres which are smaller in diameter than the rest of the myocardium.

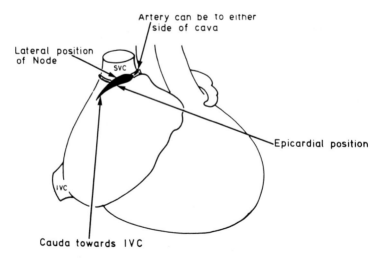

Fig. 12. *Diagram illustrating the blood supply of the sinus node.*

There are numerous nerve endings in the node: the parasympathetic fibres being derived from the right vagus. The blood supply is varied. A single artery, the nodal artery, is often found extending throughout the length of the node (see Fig. 12).

INTERNODAL TRACTS

Much controversy exists regarding the nature of these tracts. Recently James (1966) has postulated that special pathways exist in the atrium, linking the sinus and atrioventricular nodes. However, there is *no* evidence of histologically specialized internodal pathways, the conduction occurring preferentially along the thick muscle bundle of the right atrium. (*Janse and Anderson 1974*)

ATRIOVENTRICULAR JUNCTION

Atrioventricular (A-V) node

The A-V node lies between the opening of the coronary sinus and the posterior border of the membranous interventricular septum. The node is divided into a transitional zone and a compact portion.

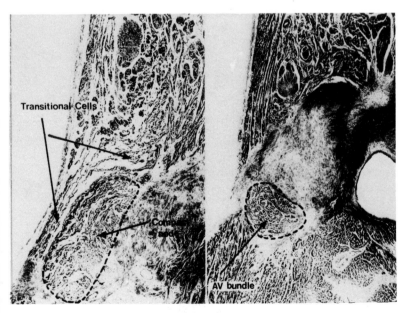

Fig. 13. (left) *Photomicrograph of the A-V node;*
(right) *Photomicrograph of the A-V bundle.*

Its important function is to cause a delay of approximately 0.04 s in A-V transmission. Two advantages result from this normal delay:

1. Postponement of ventricular excitation until the atria have had time to eject their contents into the ventricles.
2. Limit of the maximum number of signals which can be accommodated for transmission by the A-V node.

The A-V node has a similar meshwork structure to the sinus node, but there is much less collagen in the framework. In general the fibres are thicker and shorter than those of the sinus node, but not as thick as those of ordinary myocardium. There is a rich nerve supply, with the parasympathetic fibres being derived from the left vagus. The blood supply is from a specific artery, *ramus septi fibrosi*, which is a branch of the right coronary artery.

Atrioventricular (A-V) bundle (Bundle of His)

The A-V bundle extends from the A-V node through the central fibrous body from where it descends along the posterior margin of the membranous portion of the interventricular septum, to the crest of the muscular septum. Here it bifurcates into the right and left bundle branches.

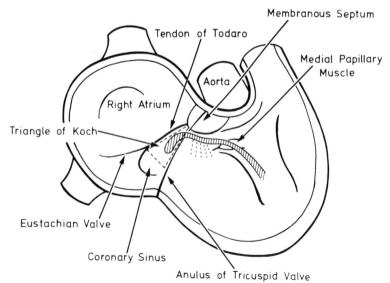

Fig. 14. *Diagram showing gross landmarks of the A-V conducting system.*

The A-V bundle is oval or triangular in cross-section. The fibres of the bundle are separated by fine collagen septums. They run parallel to one another, therefore differing from the sinus and A-V nodes, where interweaving occurs.

BUNDLE BRANCHES

The right and left bundle branches extend subendocardially along both septal surfaces.

The *right bundle branch* is a cord-like structure which passes down the side of the right ventricular septum towards the apex. It gives off few branches at first and lies more deeply beneath the endocardium than does the left main bundle. It then runs in the free edge of the moderator band to reach the base of the anterior papillary muscle where it ramifies amongst the right ventricular musculature.

The *left bundle branch* is an extensive sheet of fibres which passes down the smooth side of the left ventricular septum. The initial part of the left bundle is a continuous fan which breaks up into three interconnecting divisions: anterior, middle and posterior.

Most of the fibres in the bundle branches have thicker myofibrils with rectangular or oblong nuclei.

BLOOD SUPPLY OF HEART

CORONARY ARTERIES

The normal heart and the proximal portions of the great vessels receive their blood supply from the two coronary arteries. These arise from the *aortic bulb* which is composed of the three *aortic sinuses* (*sinuses of Valsalva*).

The *right coronary artery* arises from the right sinus of the aorta and runs forward beneath the right auricle to the atrioventricular groove. It passes downwards in the groove, embedded in fat and rounds the inferior margin of the heart, giving off its marginal branch before passing into the posterior atrioventricular groove. It then usually turns down in the interventricular groove as the *posterior interventricular branch* which descends towards the interventricular branch of the left coronary artery, supplying branches to the ventricles and interventricular septum. Frequently a *transverse branch* continues in the posterior atrioventricular groove, supplying branches to the left atrium, before anastomosing with the circumflex branch of the left coronary artery.

The *left coronary artery* arises from the left posterior sinus of the aorta and runs to the left behind the pulmonary trunk and then forwards between it and the left auricle to the atrioventricular groove. Here, it divides into its two branches; an *anterior interventricular (descending)* and a *circumflex branch*. The anterior interventricular branch descends in the anterior interventricular groove, largely embedded in fat, to the inferior margin of the heart where it turns round to ascend a short distance up the posterior interventricular groove, supplying both ventricles and the interventricular septum, anastomosing with the posterior interventricular branch of the right coronary artery. The circumflex branch passes round the left margin of the heart in the

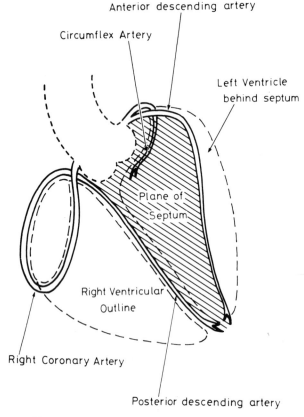

Fig. 15. *Diagram showing the coronary arteries.*

atrioventricular groove, supplying branches to the left atrium and left surface of the heart, towards the transverse branch of the right coronary artery. In some hearts the circumflex artery gives rise to the posterior descending artery. This is called left dominance.

The *left marginal branch* arises from the circumflex, and runs down the left margin of the left ventricle.

Coronary arteries only fill during ventricular diastole, and are compressed in ventricular systole.

COLLATERAL CIRCULATION

The coronary arteries are commonly subject to damage, therefore it is important to recognise the collateral circulation, both *cardiac* and *extracardiac* anastomoses.

Cardiac anastomoses. In the myocardium, there are very rich anastomoses between the right and left coronary arteries, but the vessels involved are small. These anastomoses are genetically determined and it has been shown that a gradual onset of occlusion will allow these vessels to enlarge. However, if there is a sudden occlusion, then necrosis of a segment of cardiac muscle will result.

Extracardiac anastomoses. These pass from the coronary arteries, and through the pericardium with the four pulmonary and two caval veins to anastomose with branches of the internal thoracic bronchial and phrenic arteries.

CORONARY VEINS

The veins of the heart drain chiefly into the *coronary sinus* which occupies the posterior part of the atrioventricular groove, between the left atrium and left ventricle, and opens into the right atrium.

The main tributaries of the coronary sinus are associated with the branches of the coronary arteries. The three largest are the *great* and *middle cardiac veins* and the *posterior left ventricular vein.* They may be guarded by unicuspid or bicuspid valves, which are fairly well developed. The *oblique vein of the left atrium (Marshall)* enters the sinus near the orifice of the *great cardiac vein.* It has no valve. The *small cardiac vein* may enter the right atrium directly.

One or two large *anterior cardiac veins* open directly into the right atrium. Small veins, *venae cordis minimae* (*Thebesian*) veins begin in the heart wall and open directly into the heart chambers.

BLOOD SUPPLY OF THE CONDUCTING SYSTEM

SINUS NODE

The S-A node receives its blood supply from a special artery which, in 60% of cases, arises from the right coronary artery, and in the remaining 40% of cases from the left coronary artery.

ATRIOVENTRICULAR NODE

The A-V node receives its blood supply from a specific artery, the *ramus septi fibrosi*, which arises from the right coronary artery in 90% of cases, and from the left circumflex artery in the remaining 10%.

BUNDLE OF HIS AND BUNDLE BRANCHES

The Bundle of His and the proximal few millimetres of both branches are supplied by the terminal branch of the ramus septi fibrosi from behind, and from the septal branches of the anterior descending artery.

The bundle branches are also supplied by septal arteries from the left anterior interventricular artery.

LYMPH VESSELS OF THE HEART

The heart is rich in lymphatic capillaries which form a continuous network extending throughout its mass from the endocardium to the epicardium. Large vessels form subendocardial and subepicardial plexuses. The main collecting trunks accompany the larger blood vessels in the grooves of the heart. One large trunk ascends on each side of the heart near the commencement of the corresponding artery to end in anterior mediastinal nodes, just below the arch of the aorta, and at the bifurcation of the trachea.

The final drainage is to the thoracic duct, though there may be a connection also with the broncho-mediastinal trunk on the right side.

NERVE SUPPLY OF THE HEART

Innervation of the heart is derived from the *autonomic nervous system* and contains both *sympathetic* and *parasympathetic* (*vagal*) elements which are antagonistic in function. Stimulation of the vagus results in slowing of the heart, whereas stimulation of the sympathetic results in acceleration.

Sympathetic nerve fibres supply the S-A node, atrial muscle, A-V node, specialized conduction tissue and the ventricular muscle, whereas parasympathetic fibres supply only the S-A node, atrial muscle and A-V node, and not the ventricular conduction tissue or ventricular myocardium.

In addition to their *efferent* fibres, the vagal nerves contain *afferent* fibres. The afferents transmit impulses to the central nervous system from discrete cardiac receptor endings of various types and form terminal networks in areas such as the endocardium around the openings of venae cavae, pulmonary veins, over the interatrial septum and in the atrioventricular valves. The efferents transmit impulses which are modified reflexly by afferent impulses from the heart and great vessels. They are under the overall control of the higher centres in the brain, the hypothalamus and the mid-brain.

Since the heart develops in the neck and later migrates caudally into the thorax, it therefore takes with it its original nerve supply, which consists of the *cervical cardiac branches* of the vagus and sympathetic.

The cervical branches are reinforced in the thorax by additional vagal and sympathetic nerves, and are then distributed to the heart by the *cardiac plexus* which lies between the concavity of the aortic arch and the tracheal bifurcation. The upper cervical cardiac branch of the left cervical sympathetic chain and the lower cervical branch of the left vagus pass down near the aortic arch on its left side. Entering the wall of the aorta are afferent fibres of the *pressor-receptors* which detect an increased pressure in the aorta and carotid arteries and in turn signal the cardiovascular regulatory centre of the medulla oblongata to cause slowing of the heart rate (Marey's reflex). It is thought that most of the cardiac fibres of the right vagus terminate in the sinuatrial node, while the majority of the fibres of the left vagus terminate in the atrioventricular node. Some vagal fibres probably terminate in the walls of the great veins near their entrance of the right atrium, and are responsible for the cardiac acceleration which accompanies increased venous return to the heart (Bainbridge reflex).

CHEMORECEPTORS

Chemoreceptors located in the arterial wall at the carotid bifurcation and aortic arch detect changes in blood pO_2, pCO_2, and pH. The afferent impulses arising in these fibres mainly alter respiration, but to a lesser degree modify the heart rate and vasomotor tone. The afferent impulses from the chemoreceptors pass with the afferent fibres from pressor-receptors via the IX (Glossopharyngeal) and X (Vagus) cranial nerves to the cardiovascular regulatory centre.

ELECTROPHYSIOLOGY OF THE HEART

Cardiac electrophysiology is a complex subject; a few basic principles are presented here. Electricity originates in the heart of the myocardial cells due to chemical changes taking place. Cardiac muscle consists of discrete cells of different types. The two important cell types are the *myocardial* cells and *pacemaker* or *automatic* cells.

Within these two groups there are differences; e.g. myocardial cells in the atrium are anatomically and physiologically different from the myocardial cells in the ventricle.

MYOCARDIAL CELLS

The myocardial cells are the heart muscle cells. The main bulk of the atria and ventricles consists of these cells, arranged in columns. Their function is to provide the mechanical pumping action of the heart. There are four basic elements in the myocardial cells structure:

1. *Cell membrane*
2. *Cytoplasm*
3. *Contractile elements*
4. *Sarcoplasmic reticulum*

Each cell contains a central nucleus with many myofibrils aligned along the cells axis, and a large number of mitochondria. The cell is enclosed by its membrane or sarcolemma through which the cardiac electrical activity exerts its important function.

Examined under an electron microscope the myofibrils resemble those of skeletal muscle, with sets of the proteins *actin* and *myosin* present in myofilaments which are arranged hexagonally. *Tropomyosin* and *troponin* are also present in the filaments of cardiac muscle.

In the mitochondria lying close to the myofibrils, the energy of the metabolic substrates (glucose, fatty acids, lactate and pyruvate) is converted to the terminal-bond energy of *creatine phosphate (CP)* and *adenosine triphosphate (ATP)*. The breakdown of ATP at the myofibrillar bridges release energy for the contraction of the myofibrils.

The myocardial cell membrane resembles other cell membranes. Adjacent cells are held together by a complex system of interdigititating projections — *intercalated discs*.

The sarcoplasmic reticulum consists of a series of fine branching tubes forming channels or invaginations from the surface membrane of the cell down to the contractile elements. This allows changes occurring at the cell membrane to be rapidly transmitted to the contractile elements to provide the link between the electrical and mechanical activity of the heart.

Myofibrils occupy most of each muscle fibre, which when closely examined are transversely striated. These striations are divided into bands. The deeply coloured bands are the A bands alternating with I bands. In the centre of each A band is a paler region known as the H band. In the centre of each I band is a Z line. The region between each Z line is known as a *sarcomere*.

Each myofibril contains a system of longitudinal filaments arranged in a regular pattern. In the I bands there are thin filaments composed mainly of actin, but also containing troponin and tropomyosin. These filaments are attached to a part of the Z line (Z disc) and extend into the H band where they interdigitate with a system of thicker filaments, mainly composed of myosin.

When the muscle changes in length, the thick and thin filaments slide over each other. Thus, during shortening, the I band becomes narrower but the A band remains the same width.

AUTOMATIC CELLS

The automatic cells are the specialized heart cells whose function is to regulate the contraction of the myocardial cells by providing the initial electrical stimulation. These cells are found in the sino-atrial node, in the atrioventricular node, and in the ventricular conduction system. Their contractile elements are sparser and the cells do not contribute significantly to the cardiac contraction.

Although these cells are polarized their state of polarization never remains constant. The electrical charge on the cells surface leaks away until the threshold is reached, when spontaneous complete depolarization occurs over the whole cell surface at once and spreads to adjacent fibres, whether they are myocardial cells or automatic cells. If it spreads to a myocardial cell then that cell will contract it. If it spreads to another automatic cell then that cell will be depolarized before it can discharge itself. Whichever cell reaches threshold level first will go on to complete depolarisation and discharge all the remaining automatic and all the myocardial cells. The automatic cell with the most rapid leakage rate will maintain its position as the principal pacemaking cell. Normally the principal pacemaker is located within the S-A node. (Schamroth 1976)

POLARISATION

All cells contain and are surrounded by electrolytes. The two principal ions involved are *sodium* (*Na*) and *potassium* (*K*). The cell membrane separates the intracellular fluid (rich in potassium) from the extracellular fluid (rich in sodium). In the normal resting state, the cell membrane is relatively impermeable to sodium resulting in the cell membrane being positively charged on the outside and negatively charged on the inside. An active energy-consuming 'sodium pump' pushes out any sodium that may leak inwards. The concentration of sodium on the outside of the cell membrane is 30 times greater than that on the inside. Conversely, the concentration of potassium is about 30 times greater within the cell than in extracellular fluid. This cell in the 'resting state' is said to be *polarized*. The transmembrane resting potential recorded from inside the cardiac cells is about -90mV. After excitation the polarity of the charge on the membrane is reversed and the transmembrane potential changes rapidly to about +30mV. This is due to an alteration in the cell membrane for a very short time. The subsequent voltage-time curve of the membrane *action potential* is much longer than that of nerve cells. These voltage changes are produced by electric current flow, due to the movement of ions. The inward flow of sodium produces the large rapid positive potential. The outward flow of potassium produces the smaller negative one.

Electrical changes taking place in the cell precede contraction. The membrane becomes permeable to sodium which passes into the cell while potassium leaves, thus altering the electrical state. This is said to be *depolarized*.

When the cell returns to the resting state, due to potassium gradually returning to the cell as sodium is pumped out again, it is said to be *repolarized*. However, simultaneous fluxes of *calcium (Ca)* between the cell and extracellular fluid, and within the cells, play an important role.

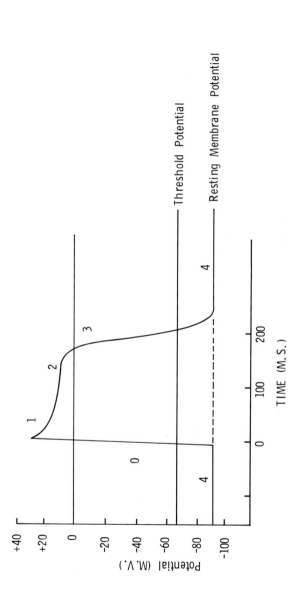

Fig. 16. *Phases of the action potential of a single myocardial cell: Phase 0: terminal phase of depolarization. Phase 1: early and rapid depolarization; Phase 2: slow repolarization (the plateau). Phase 3: terminal phase of relatively rapid repolarization. Phase 4: resting potential.*

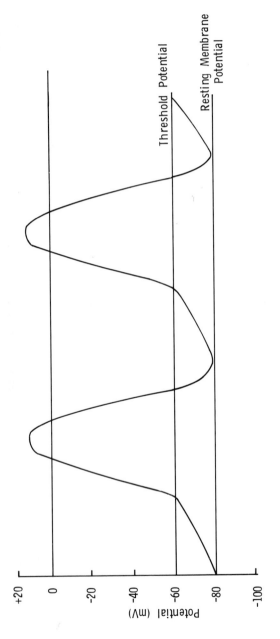

Fig. 17. *Action potential of spontaneously discharging pacemaker cell.*

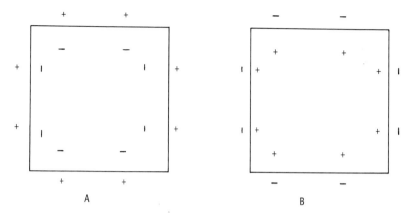

Fig. 18(a). *Diagram illustrating a polarized or resting cell.* (b) *Diagram illustrating a depolarized or activated cell.*

Once the depolarization process has started it is inevitably transmitted along the length of the cell to the next cell. In this manner a single electrical stimulus can depolarize the whole heart.

The electrical excitation of a cardiac cell membrane is due to the generation of a local circuit current by the membrane action potential. Due to positive feedback this current is responsible for the propagation of the action potential. The intercalated discs help by providing a low electrical resistance between the cells.

The membrane current is transmitted to its interior via the sarcoplasmic reticulum. Calcium is released into the myofibrils, and activates the myofilaments. The sarcomere shortens and the myofibril contracts.

PHYSIOLOGY OF THE HEART

The heart is a double pump, which maintains two circulations, the pulmonary and systemic. The heart's basic functions are to transport oxygen and other nutrients to the body cells, to remove metabolic waste products from them, and to convey substances such as hormones from one part of the body to another.

HAEMODYNAMICS

Blood entering the *right atrium* from the *superior* and *inferior venae cavae* is forced by atrial contraction through the *tricuspid valve* into the *right ventricle*. The right ventricle then pumps blood through the *pulmonary valve* into the *pulmonary artery*, thence through the lungs and finally through the *pulmonary veins* into the *left atrium*. Left atrial contraction then forces the blood through the *mitral valve* into the *left ventricle* where it is pumped through the *aortic valve* into the *aorta* and on through the systemic circulation.

The pulmonary circuit is a low pressure system with short, wide, thin walled vessels and a capacity of small volume containing at rest only 500 – 900 ml blood. Its function is to supply the lungs.

The systemic circuit is a high pressure system with long, narrow, thick walled arteries and a volume of 5 litres. Its function is to supply several regions including the coronary, cerebral, renal, hepatic and portal supplies.

THE PULMONARY CIRCUIT

The pulmonary circuit normally carries all the cardiac output through the lungs at a mean pressure in the adult of approximately 15 mmHg (less than one-sixth of that in the systemic circuit) therefore its resistance to blood flow is one-sixth of the systemic circuit. The total pulmonary blood volume is about 700 ml and, as in the systemic circulation, about 60% of this volume is on the venous side. The normal pulmonary capillary pressure is about 6 – 12 mmHg. The normal pulmonary capillary blood volume at rest is about 100 ml, less than one half that of the systemic capillaries.

THE SYSTEMIC CIRCUIT

The *aorta* functions as a compression chamber or reservoir for blood during the rapid ejection phase from the left ventricle. This is due to the elasticity of the vessel. As the branches arising from the aorta divide, the total cross-sectional area of the arteries, arterioles and capillaries increases and the average velocity of blood flow decreases. The *arterioles* offer the largest resistance to flow. The *capillaries* usually have walls consisting of single endothelial cells. In the capillary bed there is often stasis of flow in some capillaries and, at the same time, an active flow in others. The normal systemic capillary pressure is about 24 – 35 mmHg. The normal systemic capillary blood volume at rest is about 5% of the total volume (250 ml).

CORONARY CIRCULATION

About 4% of the output of the left ventricle passes into the coronary vessels. Therefore the coronary blood flow at rest is about 200 ml. About 70% of the total coronary blood flow occurs during diastole. During systole the coronary vessels lying within the heart are compressed, so that the resistance to flow at that time is sharply increased. Blood flow is largely determined by the calibre of the coronary arteries themselves.

CO-ORDINATION OF THE HEART BEAT

All cardiac muscle has the intrinsic capacity for rhythmic excitation. To prodice efficient pumping, the complex mass of myocardial fibres must contract more or less simultaneously. The ventricles are ineffective if the individual myocardial cells contract in a random fashion, e.g. in ventricular fibrillation. The atria are easily provoked into spontaneous rhythmic contraction. The ventricular muscle fibres can also contract independently, but are normally excited through the conducting tissue.

SEQUENCE OF EXCITATION

The innate rhythmiticity of cardiac muscle contraction is normally controlled by the conducting system of the heart. The anatomy of this system has already been discussed.

The sinus (S-A) node is the normal pacemaker, discharging at a more rapid rate than any other part of the conducting system. Normally, the activating impulse from the sinus node spreads in all directions. It travels at a rate of about 1 m per s, and reaches the most distant portion of the atrium in about 0.08 s, and approaches the atrioventricular (A-V) node. Here, a delay of approximately 0.04 s in atrioventricular transmission occurs. During this delay atrial systole is largely completed. After leaving the A-V node, the wave of excitement passes rapidly along the specialized fibres of the A-V bundle, bundle branches and peripheral ramifications of these branches; the spread of excitation thus causing contraction of the ventricular musculature.

THE CARDIAC CYCLE

This is the cyclical contraction (*systole*) and relaxation (*diastole*) of the two atria and the two ventricles. During diastole each chamber fills with blood, during systole the blood is expelled. Both atria and both ventricles contract almost simultaneously.

The normal heart beats about 70 times per minute in the resting adult, and the duration of the cardiac cycle is approximately 0.8 s. In the newborn infant, the cycle is of shorter duration, and the heart beats about 130 times per minute. The duration of atrial systole is approximately 0.1 s. The duration of ventricular systole is approximately 0.3 s. The duration of atrial and ventricular diastole is approximately 0.4 s.

The volume of the human heart is some 700 ml at the end of diastole, whereas the actual volume of muscle is about 300 ml. Therefore the cavities may contain about 400 ml of blood (*end-diastolic volume*), an amount that is much greater than the quantity expelled by both ventricles each time they contract (about 140 ml).

CARDIAC OUTPUT

The volume of blood pumped by the heart each minute is called the *cardiac output*. The volume ejected during systole is called the *stroke volume*. On average the adults resting stroke volume is about 70 ml. If the heart rate is 80, the cardiac output (CO is 70×80 ml; = 5600 ml per min. or 5.6 litres per min. Thus:

$$\text{CO (ml/min)} = \text{HR (beats/min)} \times \text{SV (ml/beat)}$$

The walls of the atria are thin, appropriate to the small amount of work required to force their contents into the ventricles. The thick-walled ventricles do most of the work of the heart, expelling blood into the system of branching arteries which offer considerable resistance to the onflow of blood. The wall of the left ventricle is about three times thicker than the wall of the right, appropriate to the greater amount of work performed by the left ventricle.

Control of cardiac output

To increase the cardiac output to meet the oxygem requirements, e.g. with exercise, then the heart rate or stroke volume (or both) must increase.

Heart rate. This is slowed by the vagus nerve, by releasing *acetylcholine*. It is increased by stimulation of the sympathetic nerves of the heart, releasing *noradrenaline*. Circulating *adrenaline* and noradrenaline may also increase the heart rate.

Stroke volume. This may be increased in two ways: (a) by increasing the filling of the heart; (b) by improving the efficiency of contration.

(a) Increased filling of the heart. Within certain limits, cardiac muscle fibres contract more forcibly the more they are stretched before contraction begins (*Starlings Law* of the heart). This stretching of the fibres is achieved by increasing venous return to the heart, which results in greater filling. The more forceful contraction which ensues empties the heart more efficiently, thus increasing the stroke volume.

(b) Improved efficiency of contraction. In addition to increasing the heart rate (*chronotropic effect*) the sympathetic nerves of the heart and circulating adrenaline improve the speed and strength of contraction (*inotropic effect*).

These mechanisms normally operate together to increase the cardiac output as required.

INTER-RELATIONSHIPS BETWEEN PRESSURE, FLOW AND RESISTANCE

Blood flow means simply the quantity of blood that passes a given point in the circulation in a given period of time. Flow through a blood vessel is determined by:

(a) The *pressure difference* tending to push blood through the vessel.

(b) The impediment to blood flow through the vessel, which is called vascular *resistance*.

Blood pressure means the force exerted by the blood against any unit area of the vessel wall.

Resistance is the impediment to blood flow in a vessel. It must be calculated from measurement of blood flow and pressure difference in the vessel. *Total peripheral resistance* is the resistance of the entire systemic circulation.

The amount of blood that flows into the heart each minute (venous return) and that is pumped each minute (cardiac output) is determined by:

(a) arterial pressure

(b) total peripheral resistance

When the arterial pressure remains normal, as it usually does, venous return and cardiac output are then inversely proportional to the total peripheral resistance.

NORMAL ARTERIAL BLOOD PRESSURE

Blood enters the arterial system from the left ventricle and leaves through the arterioles. The amount entering is determined by the cardiac output, and the amount leaving is determined by the peripheral resistance. If the cardiac output increases or if the peripheral resistance rises, the pressure in the arterial system rises. Conversely, if cardiac output or peripheral resistance falls, the arterial pressure decreases. Blood pressure is therefore directly proportional to cardiac output and peripheral resistance.

A normal level of pressure is maintained by reflex arcs derived from

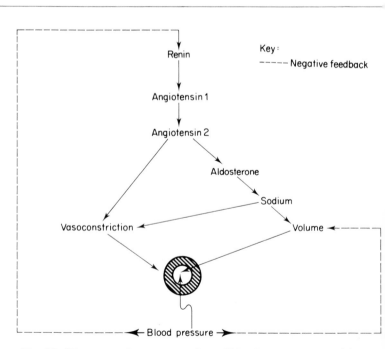

Fig. 19. *Diagrammatic representation of blood pressure control by hormonal influences.*

stretch receptors found in the wall of the proximal arterial tree, especially in the region of the aortic arch and carotid sinuses. When the arterial pressure rises there is increased stimulation of these nerve endings. The increased traffic of impulses up the vagus and glossopharyngeal nerves leads to reflex vagal slowing of the heart and reflex release of vasoconstrictor tone in the peripheral blood vessels. The resulting fall in cardiac output and the reduction of peripheral resistance tend to restore the blood pressure to the normal value. Likewise, a fall in the arterial pressure decreases the stimulation of the arterial stretch receptors. The reflex tachycardia and vasoconstriction that ensue tend to raise the blood pressure towards its normal value.

It is known that a fall in renal blood flow, due to a fall in arterial pressure results in the release of a proteolytic enzyme, renin, produced in the kidney by the juxta-glomerular apparatus (JGA). Renin converts the plasma protein angiotensinogen to the physiologically inactive polypeptide angiotensin I, further changed in the lungs to angiotensin II. This substance is a potent vasoconstrictor and it also stimulates the adrenal glands to an increased production of aldosterone. The salt and water retention brought about by aldosterone together with the vasoconstriction produced by angiotensin II tend to raise arterial pressure to the set value. (*Thompson 1981*)

SEQUENCE OF EVENTS DURING THE CARDIAC CYCLE

Provided the heart receives excitation along the normal pathways and the heart rate remains constant, each successive cardiac cycle follows the same patterns of systole and diastole.

Arterial function

In atrial systole contraction of the right atrium usually very slightly precedes that of the left. The muscular contraction forces blood from the atria through the A-V valves into the ventricles during the last phase of passive ventricular filling. This causes small increases in the pressures in both the atria and the ventricles because the A-V valves are still open. As there are no valves between the right atrium and venae cavae, some blood is expelled backwards during atrial systole into the superior vena cava, where it causes a rise both in the pressure and in the volume. At the end of atrial systole the blood continues to move through the valves because of its inertia, leaving for a short period a reduction in pressure which causes the valve cusps to close. The delay of electrical transmission at the A-V node allows the atria to contract completely before ventricular contraction starts.

Ventricular function

Ventricular systole begins soon after the start of ventricular excitation. The pressure of blood in the ventricles begins to rise while that in the relaxing atria is falling. The cusps of the A-V valves close and then bulge backwards momentarily into the atria. The surfaces of their cusps being held in apposition by the pull of the papillary muscles on the chordae tendineae attached to the cusp edges. This momentary backward bulging of the A-V valve cusps produces slight transient increases of pressure in the atria. After the closure of the A-V valves the blood pressure rises in both ventricles; because both the A-V and the semi-lunar valves are closed the volume of intraventricular blood remains constant. During this *isovolumetric* (*isometric*) phase of ventricular contraction the ventricles alter their shape, becoming plumper. When the rising ventricular pressures exceed the pressures in the aorta and pulmonary artery the semi-lunar valves open, the isometric phase ends and the ejection (*isotonic*) phase of contraction begins. At the end of this phase, the ventricular muscle relaxes, and when the pressures fall below those in the aorta and pulmonary artery, the semi-lunar valves close.

Throughout ventricular systole the ventricular volume falls. Simultaneously, blood has been entering the atria; because the A-V valves are closed the intra-atrial pressure gradually rises.

After the closure of the semi-lunar valves, the pressure in the ventricles fall rapidly and is soon below that in the atria. At this point the A-V valves open and blood flows passively from the atria to the ventricles, at first very fast, later more slowly.

Electrolytes and the heart

Electrolytes and acid-base abnormalities may exert profound effects on myocardial impulse formation, conduction, contractility, repolarization, and rhythmicity. Most of the abnormalities are functional and therefore reversible with correction of the electrolyte imbalance.

Sodium and potassium are the ions mainly responsible for myocardial activity. Myocardial fibre potentials are dependent on the potassium/sodium ratio in the fibres and/or the intracellular-extracellular gradient of these ions. The main effect of potassium is on the resting membrane potential, while sodium influences the action potential. Calcium affects myocardial contractility.

Electrolytes and acid-base imbalance in the context of cardiac arrhythmias will be discussed in the next chapter.

IMPLICATIONS FOR THE NURSE

The nurse should understand the role of the heart in the context of the person's physiology as a whole. She should comprehend the normal development, structure, and function of the heart as this will enable her to understand more clearly any subsequent pathology. For example, a knowledge of the precise location of the conducting system should be of both importance and interest to the nurse so that she more readily comprehends the basis of many of the cardiac arrhythmias she must encounter. In order to appreciate cardiac disease these principles are discussed in relation to different disorders, therefore making them more meaningful. Such appreciation will enable the nurse to understand the rationale of medical decisions and the implications of these which she may be asked to follow.

REFERENCES

Anderson, R.H. & Becker, A.E. (1980) *Cardiac anatomy: an integrated text and colour atlas.* London: Gower Press.

James, T.N. (1966) Connecting pathways between the sinus node and the A-V node and between the right and left atrium in the human heart. *Am. Heart J., 66,* 498.

Janse, M.J. & Anderson, R.H. (1974) Specialized inter-nodal atrial pathways — fact or fiction? *European Journal of Cardiology, 2,* 117.

Schamroth, L. (1976) *An introduction to electrocardiography.* Oxford: Blackwell Scientific Publications.

Shinbourne, E.A. & Anderson, R.H. (1980) *Current paediatric cardiology.* Oxford: Oxford University Press.

Starling, E.H. (1918) *The Linacre Lecture on the law of the heart.* London: Longmans, Green & Co.

Thompson, D.R. (1981). Recording patients' blood pressure: a review. *J. adv. Nurs., 6,* 283.

Thompson, D.R. & Anderson, R.H. (1982) The conduction system of the heart. *Nurs. Times, 78,* 310.

Thompson, D.R. & Anderson, R.H. (1982) The normal development of the heart. *Nurs. Times* (in press).

3
Electrocardiography

INTRODUCTION

Electrocardiography can be defined as the recording of electrical activity in the heart by recordings taken at the body surface. These may be displayed on special graph paper or on a screen to give a visual impression, e.g. an oscilloscope (monitor). An electrocardiogram (ECG) is a record of these electrical voltage variations plotted against time. An electrocardiograph machine is a galvanometer which records these voltage variations. The first such machine was developed by Wilhelm Einthoven (1903).

Electrocardiography is an essential part of the examination of the cardiovasular system, but like any other diagnostic test must be taken together with all other information. The main clinical value of the ECG is in the interpretation of cardiac arrhythmias, diagnosis of ischaemic heart disease, and in the assessment of ventricular hypertrophy.

A few basic principles of cardiac electrophysiology have already been described. So too has the conducting system of the heart and the electrical changes which take place (see p. 20). These are detected by a galvanometer, a special instrument used for measuring the strength of an electrical current. The electrodes of a galvanometer in an electrocardiograph are arranged so that when a wave of depolarization moves towards a recording electrode an upright deflection is obtained, an

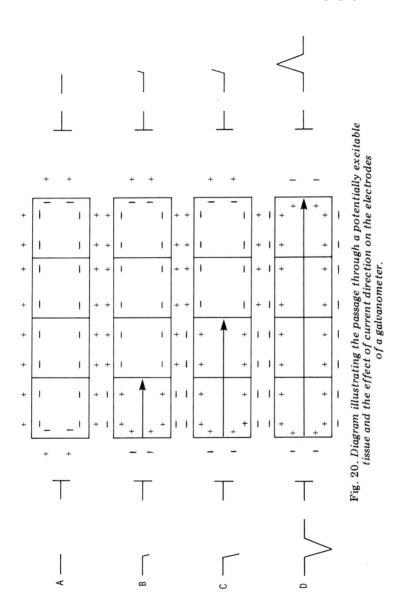

Fig. 20. *Diagram illustrating the passage through a potentially excitable tissue and the effect of current direction on the electrodes of a galvanometer.*

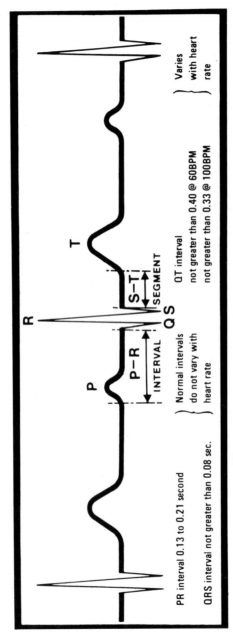

Fig. 21. Representation of a normal electrocardiogram.

electrode of the opposite side of the body shows a downwards deflection. The sequence of waves produced at each heart beat has been labelled P, Q, R, S, T and U.

The P wave is associated with atrial activation, the QR and S wave with ventricular activation and the T and U waves with ventricular recovery.

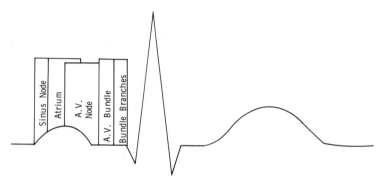

Fig. 22. *Diagrammatic representation of activation sequences of the separate regions within the P-R interval.*

DEFINITIONS OF THE DEFLECTIONS

The P Wave:
This is a blunt upright deflection not more than 2.5 mm in amplitude and 0.08 s in duration. It precedes the QRS complex.

The QRS complex:
The Q wave: This is the first downward deflection which is followed by an upward one. If no upward deflection is present a downward deflection is called QS.

The R wave: This is the first upward deflection.

The S wave: This is a downward deflection which follows an R wave.

The ST segment: This is a nearly horizontal (iso-electric) segment between the end of the QRS and the beginning of the T wave.

The T Wave:
This is a broad, blunt deflection arising from the end of the ST segment. Its amplitude varies considerably and its duration varies between 0.18 – 0.20 s.

The U wave: This is a small deflection occasionally seen following the T wave.

LEAD SYSTEMS

LEADS

The standard electrocardiogram (ECG) consists of tracings from twelve or more leads. They are the three standard (bipolar) limb leads, I, II, and III; three unipolar limb leads, a VR, a VL, and a VF; and six unipolar chest leads, V1 to V6.

The term 'lead' refers to the ECG obtained as a result of recording the difference in electrical potential between a pair of electrodes. All the leads record the same electrical activity of the heart, but since they view it from different positions on the body surface, the deflections are different in appearance in the various leads.

ELECTRODES

These are simply low-resistance connexions designed to sense electrical activity at the body surface. These skin electrodes may be placed on either the chest or limbs depending upon the monitoring situation. Chest electrodes are preferred, because a better signal can be obtained. The electrical changes, which are small, are transmitted, usually along wires (although radiotelemetry is gaining popularity in some centres) to amplifiers. It is then displayed on an oscilloscope (monitor), a paper chart recorder, or recorded onto magnetic tape for analysis later. Most of the electrodes now used for continuous monitoring are of the disposable type. Many of the problems associated with ECG electrodes can be prevented by using high quality electrodes, proper skin preparation technique, and correct application technique.

STANDARD (BIPOLAR) LIMB LEADS

The galvanometer of the electrocardiograph machine carries two poles or terminals. Each of these poles is connected through a lead selector switch to electrodes placed on various parts of the body. The recorded deflections represent the difference in voltage applied across these poles. Thus, the standard or bipolar leads represent differences between the limbs. Lead I equals the voltage on the left arm minus the voltage on the right (LA – RA), Lead II = LL – RA, and Lead III = LL – LA. The zero points are located midway between the extremities. The limbs behave simply as conductors away from the trunk. The left leg functions as the inferior angle of an equilateral triangle in the frontal plane.

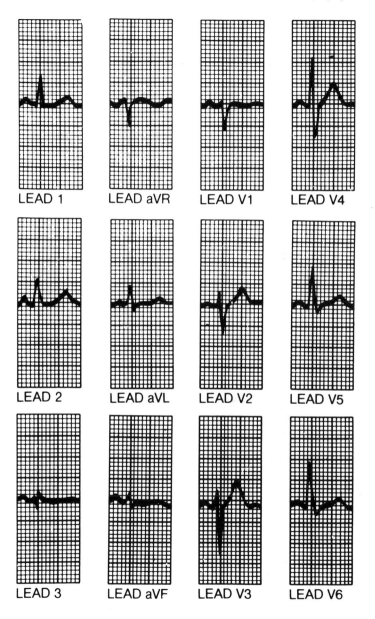

Fig. 23. *Electrocardiogram of a normal heart.*

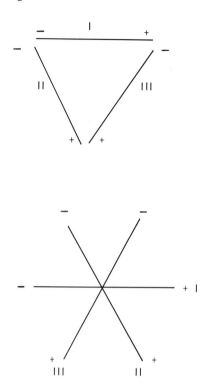

Fig. 24. *Diagram of the bipolar (standard) leads.*

If the sides of the triangle are displaced centrally but parallel to their normal positions, so that their zero points coincide, it will be seen that Lead I occupies a horizontal position running between $0°$ on the left and $180°$ on the right intersection with a circle inscribed around the original triangle. Lead II runs between $+60°$ at its positive end and $-120°$ on the negative; Lead III is positive at $+120°$ and negative at $-60°$. The galvanometer is arranged to record an upstroke if the potential at the positive pole exceeds that of the negative pole.

UNIPOLAR LIMB LEADS

In these leads the galvanometer is arranged to record the potential variations on each limb separately instead of recording the algebraic sum of two as in the standard leads. One pole of the galvanometer is

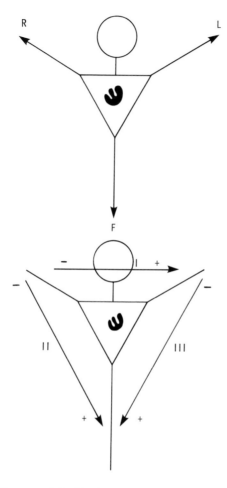

Fig. 25. *Diagram of the bipolar (standard) and unipolar leads.*

connected to a central terminal which is connected to all three limbs. The sum of the potential variations of these three limbs is zero, so that the central terminal is zero. This corresponds to the centre of the chest and coincides with the conjunction of the zero points of the bipolar leads. The other pole of the galvanometer is connected in turn to each of the three limbs. The three unipolar limb leads are VR (right arm), VL (left arm), and VF (left leg or foot). V stands for voltage. The voltages recorded are very low and so are increased (augmented) to

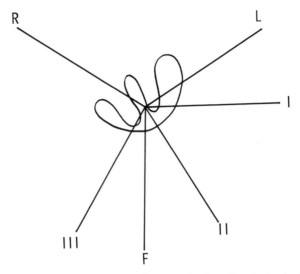

Fig. 26. *Diagram of the bipolar (standard) and unipolar leads.*

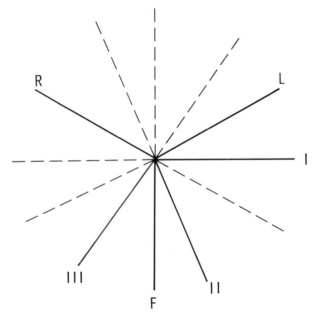

Fig. 27. *Diagram of the bipolar (standard) and unipolar leads in relation to the hexaxial reference system.*

make them comparable with those from other leads; they are therefore designated aVR, aVL, and aVF.

In effect, the three standard and the three unipolar limb leads arranged in the frontal plane with coinciding zero points constitute a hexaxial reference system with six dimensions, six positive and six negative ends (each at a distance of 30° away).

UNIPOLAR CHEST (PRECORDIAL) LEADS

These leads are influenzed by electrical activity throughout the whole heart, but especially by the area of the heart nearest to the electrode. Owing to the close proximity of an electrode to the heart, the changes in electrical potential are greater than those recorded in the limb leads.

The chest leads are positioned as follows:

V1: Fourth intercostal space just to the right of the sternum.
V2: Fourth intercostal space just to the left of the sternum.
V3: Midway between V2 and V4 positions.
V4: Fifth interspace in left midclavicular line.
V5: Directly lateral to V4 in the left anterior axillary line.
V6: Directly lateral to V4 and V5 in the left mid-axillary line.
In females, the left-sided leads are placed under not over the left breast.

These six unipolar leads provide detailed information about the heart. V1 and V2 face the free wall of the right ventricle, V3 and V4 are opposite the interventricular septum, and V5 and V6 face the free wall of the left ventricle.

Additional recordings can be taken from V3R and V4R — sites on the right side of the chest equivalent to V3 and V4. Recordings may also be taken at higher levels, e.g. second, third or fourth spaces or further laterally (V7 and V8).

CARDIAC VECTORS

A vector is a term used in physics to express the magnitude and direction of an electrical force in the three places of space. The heart can be thought of as a source of electromotive force in the centre of an equilateral triangle. The portion of the electrical vector recorded in an individual lead depends on the angle between the vector and the direction of the lead; if the vector is parallel to the lead it will be fully recorded in that lead; if the vector is perpendicular to the direction of the lead, no potential difference will be recorded in that lead. If the vector is intermediate to those previously stated, a corresponding vector will be recorded in that lead.

The total electrical activity at any one time can be summated and represented as the *instantaneous vector*. All the instantaneous vectors occurring throughout the cardiac cycle form the *cardiac vector*.

The mean frontal plane QRS axis

The cardiac vector is described as the mean QRS vector or axis. It is customary to measure the mean QRS axis in the frontal plane. To describe the axis more precisely, the hexaxial reference system is used.

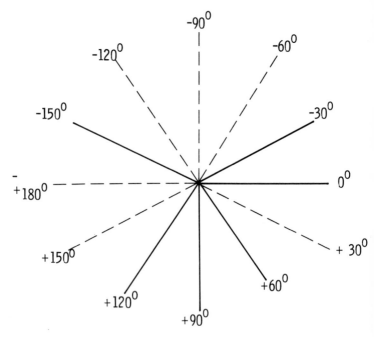

Fig. 28. *The hexaxial reference system.*

If the six limb leads (I, II, III, aVR, aVL, and aVF) are produced through their centres there are then twelve leads each at 30° to the adjacent lead. A method of determining the mean QRS axis is to inspect the six frontal plane limb leads to find the one in which the algebraic sum of all deflections within a QRS complex is most nearly equal to zero (i.e. all negative deflections are subtracted and all positive deflections are added). It is convenient to use the small squares on the ECG paper for doing this. The smallest mean QRS deflection will always be in a lead at right angles to the axis. For example, if the lead showing the smallest net QRS size is Lead II, then the lead at right angles is Lead aVL. The axis must then be directly along the lead (in this case aVL), or directly away from it, both of these positions being a right angles to the lead with the smallest net QRS size (in this case II). To determine which of these two possibilities is correct, the ECG is inspected (in lead aVL). The QRS must have a large dominant positive wave, or alternatively a large dominant negative wave. If the former, the axis of the heart is along the lead (aVL), if the latter the axis is directed away from the lead.

The normal range for the mean frontal plane QRS axis in adults is from $-30°$ to $+90°$. Axes more negative than $-30°$ are described as left axis deviation. Axes more positive than $+90°$ are described as right axis deviation.

VECTORCARDIOGRAPHY

The vectorcardiogram (VCG) is capable of plotting the forces of the cardiac vectors in two directions simultaneously. It represents the ECG as a three dimensional loop. These *vector loops* can be obtained in frontal, horizontal and sagittal planes. A three-lead system is used for recording based on a left, X, an inferior, Y, and an anterior lead, Z. The vector loop usually consists of a series of dots placed 2 m.s. apart.

Used in conjunction with a computer, it is possible to record the magnitude of the spatial vector as well as the projection in the different planes.

Vectorcardiography is technically more complex than conventional (scalar) electrocardiography.

RECORDING TECHNIQUE

The body fluids are a very good conduction system, allowing electrical changes to be detected by electrodes placed on the body surface.

Before recording starts the patient needs to be told what is involved in clear, simple terms. It should be explained that the machine will not cause any harm. He should not be unduly anxious and should prefer-ably be comfortable and relaxed; any fine muscle tremor may distort

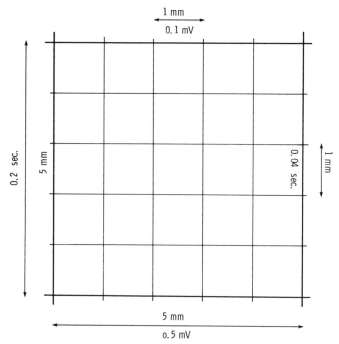

Fig. 29. *Diagram of ECG recording paper.*

the ECG record. Check for any electrical equipment nearby that may cause electrical interference.

The electrode leads (which are correctly labelled) are attached to the patients limbs and chest, after a special conducting gel has been applied to the skin surface (shaved if necessary and clean and dry).

If the ECG machine is not automatically calibrated it must be adjusted so that a vertical deflection of 1 cm is produced by a current of 1 mV.

The special ECG recording graph paper is divided into 5 mm squares by bold lines, subdivided into 1 mm squares by feint lines. The paper moves under the recording pen at a speed of 25 mm per second. Therefore one large square is equal to 0.2 s and 1 mV is equal to a deflection of 1 cm (two large squares).

Voltage of upright deflections is measured from the upper border of the baseline (iso-electric line) to the peak of the wave. Downward deflections are measured from the lower border of the baseline to the lowest point (nadir) of the wave.

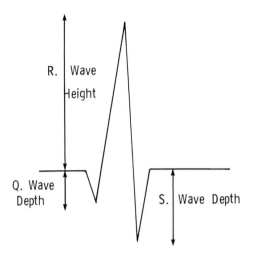

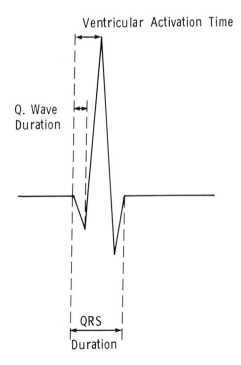

Fig. 30. *Diagram illustrating various electrocardiographic measurements.*

Abnormalities of the P wave

Right atrial hypertrophy. This causes tall, pointed P waves exceeding 2.5 mm in amplitude.

Left atrial hypertrophy. This causes prolonged and bifid P waves exceeding 0.11 s in duration.

Dextrocardia. This causes inverted P waves in leads in which they are usually upright.

Atrial ectopic beat. This causes P waves of abnormal shape, appearing earlier than the next expected normal P wave, usually followed by a normal QRS complex.

Junction rhythm. This causes inverted P waves before, during or after the QRS complex.

Sino-atrial block. This causes an absence of a PQRST complex.

Abnormalities of the P-R interval

The P-R interval is measured from the beginning of the P wave to the beginning of the QRS complex. If a Q wave is present the interval measured should be the P-Q. The normal duration of the P-R interval is 0.12 – 0.20 s.

First-degree A-V block. The P-R interval exceeds 0.20 s in duration.

Second degree A-V block (Wenckebach type). The P-R interval becomes progressively more prolonged from beat to beat until one P wave is not succeeded by a QRS complex.

Wolff–Parkinson–White Syndrome (Pre-excitation syndrome). The P-R interval is shortened probably due to the presence of an accessory conducting pathway between the atria and the ventricles.

Abnormalities of the QRS complex

The left ventricle is the greatest mass of heart muscle and dominates the ECG. If an electrode is placed over this area (lead V6) the P wave will occur, due to atrial activity. Because the first part of the ventricle to be activated is the interventricular septum from the left bundle, a Q wave will follow due to the electrical force moving away from the electrode.

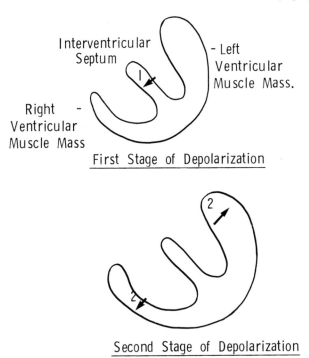

First Stage of Depolarization

Second Stage of Depolarization

Fig. 31. *Stages of ventricular depolarization.*

When the mass of the ventricle is activated the wave of excitation moves towards the electrode resulting in a positive deflection — the R wave.

If an electrode is placed over the right side of the heart (Lead V1) then a small R wave ensues, due to the spread of excitation moving towards the electrode across the septum. A negative deflection (S wave) occurs as the main muscle mass is depolarized, the bigger left ventricle (where depolarization is spreading away) outweighing the effect of the right ventricle (where depolarization is spreading towards the electrode.)

As the left ventricle dominates the right ventricle it will effect the ECG; therefore in V1 the main QRS deflection is negative whereas that in V6 is positive.

Right ventricular hypertrophy. This shows right axis deviation (the effect of right ventricular hypertrophy is to swing the average direction of the depolarization wave to the right). The leads facing the right ventricle (e.g. V1) show dominant R waves instead of the usual S waves. ST depression and T wave inversion may occur in leads with tall R waves.

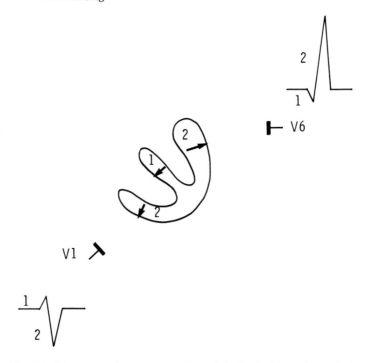

Fig. 32. *Diagrammatic representation of the basic form of ventricular depolarization and its effect on leads V1 and V6.*

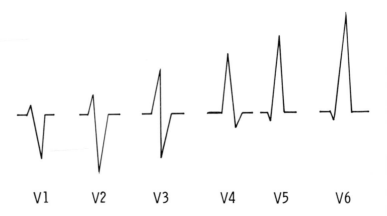

Fig. 33. *Diagrammatic representation of the precordial, chest or V leads.*

Left ventricular hypertrophy. This shows left axis deviation (the depolarization wave takes an abnormal pathway over the ventricles due to fibrosis and hypertrophy of the ventricular muscle). The hypertrophied muscle produces a larger than normal depolarization wave which is recorded as a QRS of normal configuration but increased amplitude. ST depression and T wave inversion may be present.

Right bundle branch block. The right branch of the bundle is blocked, but the septum is activated from left to right, as in the normal heart. The left ventricle is depolarized before the right. This produces a further R wave (known as R') in the right chest leads. An M pattern is thus seen in leads such as V1. The QRS usually exceeds 0.12 s in duration (normal QRS complex does not exceed 0.10 s in duration).

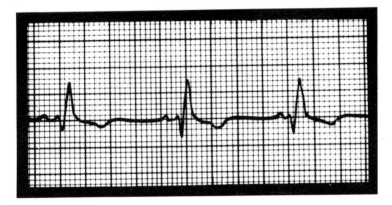

Fig. 34. *Right bundle branch block.*

Left bundle branch block. The left branch of the bundle is blocked, so the interventricular septum is activated from the right side instead of from the left. This results in the normal Q wave in the left ventricular leads being replaced by a small R wave. Right ventricular depolarization produces an R in V1 and an S in V6. When the left ventricle is depolarized an R' occurs in V6 and a broad S in V1. Thus the QRS duration exceeds 0.12 s.

Abnormalities of the ST segment
Normally the ST segment is iso-electric, but slight ST elevation may be present in the right chest leads, but not exceeding 2.0 mm. It is never

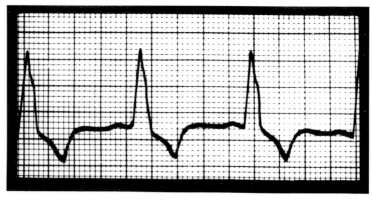

Fig. 35. *Left bundle branch block.*

normally depressed more than 0.5 mm. The point of junction between the S wave and the ST segment is known as the J point.

Acute epicardial ischaemia. This produces ST elevation. The T wave is flattened then inverted before the ST segment returns to normal.

Pericarditis. This shows ST elevation in all leads (unlike the localised changes in myocardial infarction). The T waves are low but upright and do not invert until the ST segment has returned to the iso-electric level.

Ventricular hypertrophy. This shows ST depression in the lead with the tallest R waves, sometimes with T wave inversion.

Bundle branch block. This shows ST depression in the leads with the tallest slurred R waves, with T wave inversion.

Digitalis. This shows ST depression beginning at its junction with the T wave, so that there is gentle sagging. The T wave remains upright or flattened.

Abnormalities of the T wave
Hypokalaemia. This shows a low terminal portion of the ST segment and the upstroke of the T wave.

Intracranial lesions. These may show sharply pointed T waves resembling those of ischaemic heart disease.

DISORDERS OF HEART AND RHYTHM

THE NORMAL HEART RATE AND RHYTHM

In health, the activity of the whole heart is controlled by the sinus node. The rate of discharge of the sinus node is varied by both nervous and humoral influences. The parasympathetic nerves (Vagus) decelerate, and the sympathetic nerves accelerate, the rate of the heart.

The average heart rate in healthy adults is about 72 beats per minute, but ranges between 50 and 100 per minute. The average rate in women is about 10 beats per minute more, and it is much faster in infants and young children. Lower ranges of normality are found in elderly subjects and in athletes, in whom the resting rate is commonly as low as 50 per minute. During sleep the average rate is commonly about 60 per minute. Tachycardia may occur physiologically due to increased sympathetic activity on emotion, when it commonly reaches 120 per minute; on maximum physical exercise or sexual intercourse when rates of 170 per minute may be reached. In all instances, the rhythm is perfectly regular and the JVP, pulse and heart sounds are all normal.

In children, young adults and the elderly, there is a phasic change with respiration called sinus arrhythmia. In apparently normal subjects it has been possible to analyze continuous records over periods of 24 hours or more. From these records it has been shown that abnormalities of rhythm including supraventricular tachycardia and nodal (junctional) rhythm occur quite frequently.

ARRHYTHMIAS

The normal electrocardiogram consists of a repetitive series of P, Q, R, S and T waves, which conform to established standards for shape and size, occurring 60 – 100 times per minute. In this condition, the heart is in normal sinus rhythm. This is the most effective form of myocardial contraction. (*Thompson 1979*)

The term arrhythmia is used to describe abnormalities of rate or rhythm due to the origin of impulses from an abnormal ectopic focus or to abnormal transmission of a normally arising impulse. Arrhythmias can be associated with a reduction in cardiac efficiency and may be precipitated by many causes, including myocardial infarction, hypoxia and drug toxicity (for example, with digoxin).

There are many arrhythmias, some more important than others. Common ones encountered by the nurse are presented here. The single chest lead normally used for ECG monitoring is usually sufficient for recognizing most disorders of rate and rhythm. However, it is occasionally inadequate — for example, in showing the P wave. If there is any doubt regarding a rhythm (or conduction) disturbance, a 12 lead ECG should be obtained.

Ectopic foci

Abnormal foci in the heart may produce isolated or rhythmic impulses which affect the normal heart rhythm. They may occur spontaneously or due to localised myocardial anoxia.

Re-entry

Re-entry describes the return of an impulse to an area of myocardium previously stimulated by the same impulse. This impulse may stimulate an area which is receptive but cannot activate those areas which are completely refractory. When an area recovers, it may accept the impulse and act as a pathway back to the area that was initially activated. If this latter area has had time to recover, it can be stimulated again and re-entry occurs. This process may be repeated endlessly at high speed. Re-entry in small areas of atrial (or less commonly, ventricular) muscle is known as micro re-entry, and leads to fibrillation. A long re-entrant pathway (macro re-entry) occurs if there is an accessory bundle of conducting tissue between the atrium and the ventricles as in the pre-excitation syndrome. (*Barold & Coumel 1977*)

ELECTROLYTES AND CARDIAC ARRHYTHMIAS

Potassium

The effects of *hyperkalaemia* on cardiac muscle may result in cardiac arrest. The earliest ECG changes are peaking of the T waves. However, very tall T waves are not specific for hyperkalaemia and may occur in normal individuals. As the severity of the hyperkalaemia increases, the QRS complex blends into the T wave. The P wave decreases in voltage, and may disappear entirely. With advanced hyperkalaemia, repolarization begins while some areas of myocardium are still being depolarized: producing a progressively widened QRS complex which merges into the T wave. Supra-ventricular tachycardia, ventricular ectopic beats, or atrial fibrillation may occur. In severe cases, ventricular fibrillation or asystole may ensue. (*Olsson 1980*)

Hypokalaemia also impairs myocardial contractility. ECG changes are reversed by potassium administration. The changes are flattening or inversion of the T wave, but at the same time a prominence of the U wave occurs. A low atrial muscle potassium content appears responsible for the occurrence of atrial fibrillation. Thiazide diuretics cause hypokalaemia and depletion of body potassium. Also, the more profound hypokalaemia, the greater the propensity for the occurrence of ventricular ectopic beats. (*Hollifield and Slaton 1980*)

Calcium

Hypercalcaemia increases myocardial contractility. The ECG shows a short P-R interval and a long QRS complex. The T wave begins almost immediately after the QRS complex.

Hypocalcaemia depresses myocardial contractility.

Plasma calcium levels are important in regulating cardiac excitability and myocardial contractility. It is important that great care is taken in distinguishing between hypocalcaemia and hypercalcaemia.

Magnesium

A magnesium deficiency is known to predispose to the evolution of cardiac arrhythmias (mainly ventricular ectopic beats), and an increased sensitivity to digitalis induced arrhythmias has also been shown. (*Seller et al 1970*).

Acidosis and alkalosis

The incidence of arrhythmias and the mortality rate are significantly greater in patients with severe acidosis or hypoxia. Intracellular pH changes with a change in the acid-base balance may alter myocardial contractility. Acidosis depresses myocardial function more profoundly than does alkalosis, lowering the threshold for ventricular fibrillation. (*Pilcher and Nagle 1971*).

CARDIAC ARRHYTHMIAS

Sinus rhythm

Normal cardiac activity starts in the sinus node by virtue of the fact that its rate of spontaneous depolarization is faster than that of other automatic cells. This is called sinus rhythm. The P-R interval is normal and does not alter. The QRST complexes are all identical in a given lead.

The normal heart rate in infancy is about 130 on average, and is about 72 in adults.

ECG   This shows that the P waves are normal.

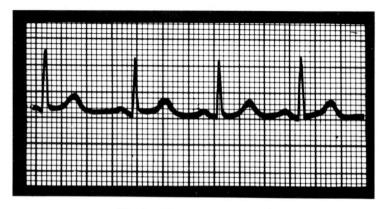

Fig. 36. *Normal sinus rhythm.*

There is one P wave to each QRS complex.
The QRS complex is normal and regular.
The P-R interval is normal and regular.

Sinus arrhythmia

Sinus heart rate increases during inspiration and slows during expiration. This is due to fluctuations in vagal tone, mediated refluxly by these phases of respiration. It is a normal phenomenon marked in the young and in people with high vagal tone.

Sinus arrhythmia is usually absent in large atrial septal defects because the venous return is not significantly affected by respiratory events.

ECG. Phasic increase/decrease occurs in the P-P interval in time with respiratory events.

Sinus tachycardia

The heart rate exceeds 100 per minute at rest, remaining under the control of the sinus node.

Causes include:

Exertion, e.g. anxiety states (or cardiac neurosis)
Thyrotoxicosis
Cardiac failure
Acute cor pulmonale

Acute pulmonary embolism
Anaemia
Blood loss
Sympathomimetic drugs (agents such as atropine sulphate)
Fever

Treatment. Sinus tachycardia is usually a physiological response to other disease or stimuli and, therefore, treatment of the arrythmia means treatment of the cause. When the response is inappropriate — as in anxiety states — or itself deleterious — as in thyrotoxicosis — specific symptomatic treatment, such as the administration of beta blocking drugs, may be advantageous.

ECG. This shows normal P waves followed by a QRS, with a fast heart rate, exceeding 100 per minute.

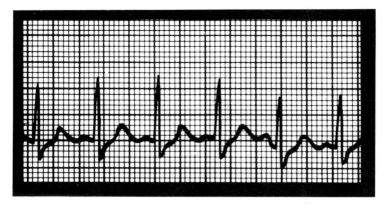

Fig. 37. *Sinus tachycardia.*

Sinus bradycardia
The heart rate is under 60 per minute at rest, remaining under the control of the sinus node.

Causes include:

Increased vagal tone
Athletic training
Increased intracranial pressure
Hypothyroidism

Digitalis therapy
>   by direct action on the sinus node (toxic effect) and
>   by increased vagotonia (therapeutic effect)

Beta-receptor blocking drugs

Organic heart disease: myocardial infarction.

Obstructive jaundice : due to bile salts' direct action on the sinus node.

Treatment. Treatment is atropine sulphate, which increases the heart rate by blocking the slowing action of the vagus nerve.

ECG. This shows normal P waves and a normal P-R interval occurring at a rate less than 60 per minute. Each P wave is followed by a QRS.

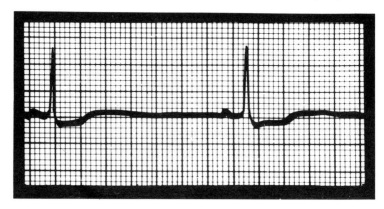

Fig. 38. *Sinus bradycardia.*

Atrial tachycardia

This occurs when an irritable focus in the atrium develops a spontaneous rate faster than the sinus node and thus assumes the pacemaker function. Though arbitrary, the rate one usually attributes to an atrial tachycardia is 140 – 220 per minute. The patient may be well aware of this sudden heart rate change. The ventricles may respond to each atrial impulse, or block may occur; the ventricles then responding to every other impulse (2:1 heart block). The duration of the arrhythmia may be seconds, minutes, hours or even weeks. Because the atrial discharge arises from a place other than the sinus node, the P wave is unusual in direction and shape. The second most common result of digoxin toxicity is atrial tachycardia with 2:1 block.

Causes include:

> Myocardial infarction or ischaemia
> Digitalis toxicity
> Heart failure

Treatment. Treatment is essential as the rapid ventricular rate increases the oxygen requirement of the myocardium. Attacks may be stopped abruptly by carotid sinus massage (CSM), however, extreme caution must be used as the effects of CSM may give rise to spontaneous symptoms of faintness or loss of consciousness. Digoxin may be given intravenously, which may convert it to a 2:1, 3:1 atrioventricular block, or alternatively beta-blocking drugs. However, it must be remembered that atrial tachycardia with a 2:1 block is the second most common result of digoxin toxicity. If these drugs are ineffective and hypotension or shock is present, then DC cardioversion to sinus rhythm is indicated.

ECG. Atrial tachycardia can easily be missed. For example, if a P wave is superimposed on the T wave, then it can easily be mistaken for a bizarre T wave. Therefore, scrutiny of T waves in suspect atrial tachycardia must be emphasized.

> P waves are abnormal.
> There must be one QRS to each P wave or to every alternate P wave (that is, there may be 2:1 atrioventricular block).
> QRS complexes are normal.

Atrial flutter

The atrial rate is about 240 - 360 per minute and the arrhythmia has the same clinical features and significant as atrial tachycardia. It is associated with a 30% reduction in cardiac output. The very rapid wide and bizarre P waves merge with each other and produce the characteristic saw-tooth appearance seen in some of the ECG leads. These special P waves are known as flutter or F waves as opposed to f waves in atrial fibrillation. The ventricles are incapable of responding to every F wave because of their rapid rate, so that some degree of atrioventricular block is inevitable; that is, 2:1 and 3:1 block.

It must be realised that atrial flutter can only be distinguished by electrocardiography. It is less common than atrial fibrillation.

Treatment. Treatment may consist of digoxin primarily, or electro-conversion by DC countershock to restore sinus rhythm. It should preferably be of low voltage (about 20 joules).

ECG. Shows that there is no iso-electric interval between adjacent P waves giving rise to a characteristic saw-tooth appearance.

Atrioventricular block is present, that is, 2:1, 3:1, 4:1 or higher. This block may be variable, thus the ventricular response (QRS) is correspondingly variable; a regular irregularity.

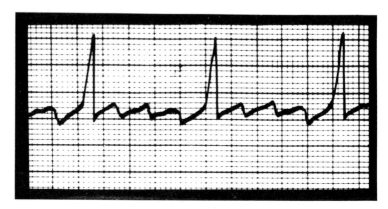

Fig. 39. *Atrial flutter.*

Atrial fibrillation

This common arrhythmia is characterised by ectopic atrial activity occurring at a very fast rate (in excess of 400 per minute), and is totally irregular. Due to some degree of atrioventricular block, the ventricular rate is usually somewhere between 100 and 150 per minute, but may range from 70 - 200 per minute.

Causes include:

Acute myocardial infarction
Rheumatic heart disease
Thyrotoxicosis
Atrial fibrillation (AF) occurs in some 15% of cases of myocardial infarction but it is usually transient.

Treatment. Treatment is conditioned by the circulatory effects of the arrhythmia. When the ventricular rate is fast and may precipitate cardiac failure, digoxin should be administered. Beta-blocking drugs may be of value. DC countershock maybe used alternatively. When the rate is relatively slow, no treatment may be required.

ECG. This shows low irregular waves (f waves) disturbing the base line. The R-R intervals are totally irregular, but the QRST complexes usually do not differ in appearance from those seen when the rhythm was sinus in origin.

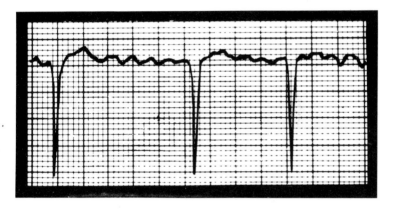

Fig. 40. *Atrial fibrillation.*

Atrial ectopic beats (synonyms: atrial extrasystole, atrial premature beat)

An atrial ectopic beat (AEB) occurs when a discharge from an ectopic atrial focus occurs prematurely. It is in some way precipitated or forced by the preceding sinus beat. AEBs may occur singly, in short runs, or intermittently.

Causes include:

Myocardial infarction
Heart failure

Treatment. No specific treatment is required. AEBs are of little importance generally but they may trigger off atrial tachycardia, atrial flutter or atrial fibrillation.

ECG. Shows the P wave occurring earlier than would be anticipated for a sinus beat, and it may be different in configuration from a P wave of sinus origin. The P-R interval in atrial ectopic beats is more often longer or at least the same as in associated conducted sinus impulse. The QRST complex may occasionally be slightly broadened and deformed in shape (aberrant).

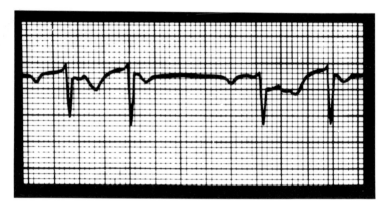

Fig. 41. *Atrial ectopic beats.*

Junctional rhythm (synonym: nodal rhythm)

The term 'junctional' is preferable to 'nodal' as it is often impossible to ascertain whether the pacemaker function is precisely originating from the atrioventricular node.

The atrioventricular junction has the ability to act as a pacemaker and normally would discharge at a rate of about 50 per minute, provided the sinus node was not discharging at a faster rate. The atrioventricular junction may become the pacemaker if the rate of discharge from the sinus node is slowed, or if the discharge rate of the junction is increased. Sometimes the junctional discharge rate is increased to 60 – 70 per minute (accelerated junctional rhythm). This is usually transient but recurrent and is often associated with atrioventricular dissociation (AVD). In junctional rhythm, the atria may or may not be activated retrogradely (i.e. with impulses of atrioventricular junctional origin).

Causes include:

Digitalis toxicity
Myocardial infarction

Treatment. Treatment is not generally required for junctional rhythm as it is a relatively benign and usually well-tolerated arrythmia. However, if the heart rate is below 50 per minute, atropine sulphate may be required.

ECG. This shows that the P waves (if present) are usually inverted. These P waves may precede, coincide or follow the QRS complex.
P waves may be absent.
QRS complexes are normal.

Junctional tachycardia (synonym: nodal tachycardia)

This is a junctional rhythm with a regular rate of 100 – 180 per minute. It is usually of a sudden onset (of which the patient may be aware). It is often paroxysmal and potentially dangerous because of the rapid rate and reduced cardiac output. Junctional tachycardia resembles atrial tachycardia, but is uncommon in acute myocardial infarction.

Causes include:

Local ischaemia of the atrioventricular junction.
In junctional rhythm, the P waves are rarely visible, except on oesophageal or atrial records.

Treatment. Treatment of this arrhythmia is required and may take the form of carotid sinus massage (CSM), or digoxin. Alternatively, beta-blocking drugs may be of use. If the arrhythmia persists, DC counter-shock should be administered.

ECG. This shows that the P waves (if visible) are abnormal in direction, for example, may be inverted.
P waves may precede, coincide or follow the QRS complex.
QRS complexes are normal in shape.

Junctional ectopic beats (synonyms: junctional, or nodal, extra-systoles; junctional, or nodal, premature beats)

Junctional ectopic beats closely resemble atrial ectopic beats, except that they originate in the atrioventricular junction. The impulse spreads into the atrium in the opposite direction from normal (thus resulting usually in inverted P waves in the ECG). The QRS complex is often aberrant, making differentiation from ventricular ectopic beats difficult.

Causes include:

Coronary artery disease
Rheumatic valvular disease

Treatment. No treatment is required.

ECG. This shows that the P waves (if visible) are inverted (especially in leads I and II). The P-R interval is abnormally short.
The P waves may precede, coincide, or follow the QRS complex.
The QRS complexes are aberrant.

Ventricular tachycardia
This is a serious rhythm disturbance, and is often preceded by ventricular ectopic beats. The ventricular rate is 120 – 200 per minute, due to an irritable focus in the ventricles (therefore taking over from the sinus node). Ventricular tachycardia is particularly serious as it may lead to ventricular fibrillation.

Causes include:

Myocardial infarction
Myocarditis
Toxic drugs (cardiac glycosides, chloroform)
Heart surgery

Treatment. Treatment is usually a bolus intravenous injection of ligno-

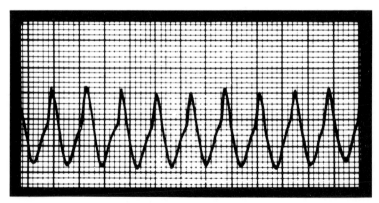

Fig. 42. *Ventricular tachycardia.*

caine (75 – 100 mg), followed by a continuous infusion. If this fails to restore sinus rhythm, DC countershock is administered (unless digitalis is implicated in the causation of the arrhythmia). When the arrhythmia ends, continuous suppressive therapy must be administered, for example, lignocaine infusion for 24 – 48 hours and oral anti-arrhythmic therapy such as procainamide. Surgical treatment of VT may even be considered if other treatment fails. (*Spurrell and Camm 1978*)

ECG. The P waves are embodied in the rapid, large ventricular complexes and are therefore difficult to identify.
The QRS complexes are broad and bizarre and are followed by T waves pointing in the opposite direction.
The R-R intervals between adjacent complexes may not be strictly regular.

Ventricular fibrillation

This serious arrhythmia is the most common cause of sudden death. It results in irreversible death unless it is corrected within a matter of minutes. It is the most important arrhythmia encountered in acute myocardial infarction and occurs in some 10% of hospital admissions.

Causes include:

Myocardial ischaemia
Injury and electrocution

The ventricular rate is rapid and irregular at 300 – 500 per minute.

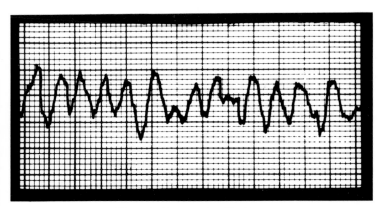

Fig. 43. *Ventricular fibrillation.*

At onset the appearance may be called ventricular flutter, as regular complexes are occurring at about 300 per minute, but they soon become faster and more irregular. Later, the complexes become flatter and eventually cardiac asystole ensues. Since there is no effective cardiac contraction, there is no cardiac output and no blood pressure. Ventricular fibrillation (VF) is thus associated clinically with cessation of the pulse, heart beat and blood pressure.

Treatment. Treatment needs to be initiated immediately, and this takes the form of DC countershock (defibrillation). If this is successful, suppressive therapy is given, for example, lignocaine infusion for 24 – 48 hours, followed by oral anti-arrhythmic therapy.

ECG. Shows broad, bizarre and irregular complexes, with no recognizable wave forms.

Ventricular ectopic beats (synonyms: ventricular extrasystole, ventricular premature beat)

Ventricular ectopic beats (VEBs) are common in acute myocardial infarction (occurring in 70 – 80% of these patients). Generally they are infrequent and of no significance. If they occur at a rate of 10 or more per minute, the prognosis is unsatisfactory, particularly when they are of the 'R on T' phenomenon. The emergence of VEBs indicates an unsatisfactory state of affairs. It is important to check that the cardiac output is not falling, that arterial oxygenation is satisfactory and that an acid-base imbalance has not developed.

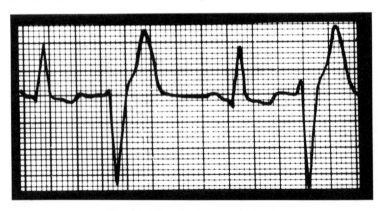

Fig. 44. *Ventricular ectopic beats.*

Causes include:

Myocardial infarction
Hypokalaemia
Digitalis
Presence of an endocardial pacemaker within the ventricle

Treatment. Treatment of VEBs is required, as they may lead on to ventricular tachycardia and ventricular fibrillation. If VEBs fall on the T wave of the previous beat ('R on T' phenomenon), this may give rise to ventricular tachycardia or fibrillation. These ectopic beats should be treated by suppressive therapy to reduce the irritability.

ECG. This shows that they occur prematurely and that the beats are not preceded by a P wave.
They are followed by a compensatory pause.
The ventricular complex is broad and bizarre, and the T wave points in an opposite direction from the main QRS deflection.

DISORDERS OF CONDUCTION

The reader is advised to read the section on the conducting system of the heart (Chapter 2), before reading this section.

Sinus arrest

This is said to occur when the regular discharge from the sinus node fails to occur or be propagated to the atrium. Because the sinus node potential is too small to be seen on the ECG, it is assumed by visible abnormalities in the ECG that when a beat is 'dropped', the P-P interval suddenly doubles. Often another focus in the atrium (the next fastest intact automatic cell) activates the heart. Because this focus may be far from the sinus node, the P wave may be deformed. The appearance and mechanism is of an escape type atrial ectopic beat.

Sinus arrest may occur with marked sinus arrhythmia and is then usually harmless. If sinus arrest is permanent and is not followed by another atrial automatic cell taking over the pacemaker function at an adequate rate, the picture is different. Under such circumstances, treatment with atropine, chronotropic agents and electrical pacing may be required.

Causes include:

> Myocardial infarction
> Digitalis intoxication

Treatment. As stated, it may require atropine sulphate, chronotropic agents or electrical pacing.

ECG. Appearance of a 'dropped' beat. The absence of a P wave can be assumed to indicate failure of the sinus node to initiate or propogate regular activity.

ATRIOVENTRICULAR BLOCK

The term atrioventricular (A-V) heart block is generally taken to refer to impaired conduction between the atrium and ventricle (atrioventricular block). This term is applied to the abnormality when the atrial impulse is delayed or completely fails to reach the ventricle. The atrioventricular junction is the most familiar site for disturbances of conduction.

It is customary and convenient to classify impaired A-V conduction into three grades:

> First degree heart block
> Second degree heart block $\Big\}$ Partial heart block
> Third degree heart block   Complete heart block

Atrioventricular block may be transient or permanent. It may be rate dependent.

Causes include:

> Congenital atrioventricular block
> Digitalis intoxication
> Myocarditis
> Idiopathic fibrosis of the conducting fibres
> Ischaemic heart disease
> Aortic valve disease

First degree A-V heart block (partial A-V heart block)
Each atrial complex is followed by a ventricular complex, but there is a delay in conduction of the impulse (leading to a prolonged P-R interval

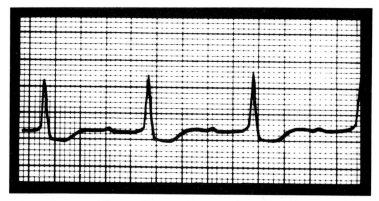

Fig. 45. *First degree A-V heart block.*

on the ECG). First degree A-V block may be the forerunner of more serious disturbances. As the block becomes progressively more severe, the conduction time is further prolonged.

Treatment. First degree A-V block requires no treatment, but the patient should be kept under close observation.

ECG. Shows a prolonged P-R interval (exceeds 0.2 s).
Normal P wave.
Normal QRST complex.

Second degree A-V heart block (partial A-V heart block)
Some atrial impulses reach the ventricles, whereas others are blocked at the atrioventricular junction.

The severity of second degree A-V block can be expressed as the ratio of the number of atrial impulses reaching the A-V junction to the number which elicit ventricular contractions. That is, it may be 5:4 or 3:2 ratio, indicating that every fifth or third impulse respectively fails to yield a ventricular response.

Two types of second degree A-V heart block are observed to occur:

Wenckebach type (Mobitz type I)
Mobitz type II

Wenckebach type (Mobitz type I) A-V block
The Wenckebach phenomenon is characterised by a progressive prolongation of the P-R interval until a ventricular complex fails to follow an

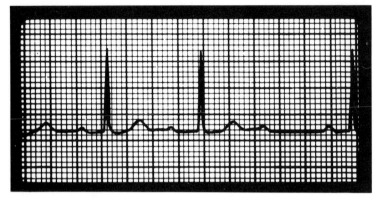

Fig. 46. *Wenckebach type (Mobitz type I) A-V heart block.*

atrial complex. Following a pause, the same cycle is then repeated.

It is usually due to a lesion involving the atrioventricular junction. As this Wenckebach phenomenon is often produced by digitalis, this should be reduced or discontinued. The patient should be closely observed due to a risk of progression to more advanced heart block.

Treatment. This arrhythmia often requires no active treatment, but the insertion of a pacing electrode into the right ventricle may be of use, so that if a more advanced degree of A-V block develops, pacing can be instituted without delay.

ECG. Shows a progressive lengthening of the P-R interval until a point is reached at which no QRS complex follows the P wave. Then the cycle repeats itself.

Mobitz type II A-V block

This is a less common type of A-V block, characterized by the sudden failure of a P wave to elicit a QRS complex without a previous warning prolongation of the P-R intervals.

This forms a striking contrast to the Wenckebach phenomenon. In its mildest form with intermittent 'dropped' beats, there is no previous prolongation of the P-R intervals, which remain normal up to the blocked beat. In more severe forms, an A-V ratio of 2:1, 3:1 or even 6:1 is obtained, the P-R interval of the conducted beat being normal.

Mobitz type II A-V block is usually associated with serious organic heart disease. It is a persistent type of A-V block and progression to

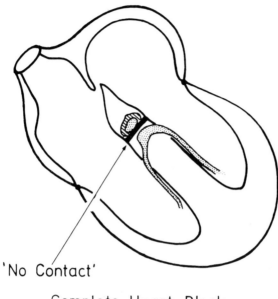

'No Contact'

Complete Heart Block

Fig. 47. *Diagrammatic representation of complete heart block.*

complete A-V block often occurs. Patients with these disturbances are liable to sudden ventricular asystole. Bradycardia is often present and may have serious effects on the circulation, for example, heart failure and cardiogenic shock. It is usually due to a lesion situated at a peripheral site in the atrioventricular junction.

Treatment. Treatment may be required if the patient is having Adams–Stokes attacks. It can take the form of an electrical pacemaking electrode connected to a demand pacemaker or an atrial triggered pacemaker. Drug therapy in the form of isoprenaline may be useful.

ECG. Shows a fixed P-R interval (which may exceed 0.2 s).
At intervals, one or more ventricular complexes are dropped.
Widening of the QRS complex may occur.

Complete A-V heart block
Complete heart block is one of the most serious complications of acute myocardial infarction. It is four times as common in men as in women.

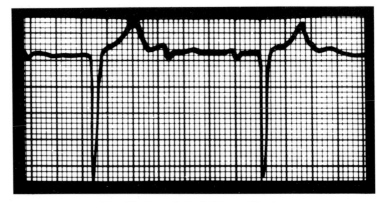

Fig. 48. *Complete A-V heart block.*

It is characterized by a failure of atrial impulses being transmitted to the ventricles, and a continued circulation is then dependent on the latter being activated by a subsidiary pacemaker. The atrial rate is faster than the ventricular rate.

Recent evidence suggests that complete heart block is commonly due to fibrosis of the conduction system, either alone or in association with diffuse myocardial fibrosis. It is most commonly a complication of occlusion of the right coronary artery which usually supplies blood to the atrioventricular junction. This artery is also responsible for supplying the inferior aspects of the heart, and a combination of complete heart block and inferior myocardial infarction is common.

Patients with complete heart block are liable to a poor prognosis as they may:

Develop complete ventricular asystole or ventricular fibrillation.

Develop extreme bradycardia which may lead to cardiac failure or shock.

Have severe myocardial damage and die even if the heart block is effectively treated.

The national mortality of complete heart block in acute myocardial infarction is about 60%, which may be reduced to about 40% by the use of drug therapy and/or pacemaking.

Treatment. Complete heart block may present as a dire emergency in acute myocardial infarction or in a patient having Adams–Stokes attacks. The choice is either drug therapy, in the form of atropine sulphate primarily and then isoprenaline; or electrical pacing, by means of a demand pacemaker.

ECG. P waves show no relationship to the QRS complexes.
QRS complexes are regular at a rate of 20 – 40 per minute.
P waves are regular at a rate of 60 – 100 per minute.

Atrioventricular dissociation

A-V dissociation is a most misunderstood term which is frequently confused with A-V block. It is important to differentiate it from A-V block as it does not have the same sinister prognosis.

Atrioventricular dissociation is a rhythm disturbance in which two separate pacemakers discharge almost simultaneously, one (usually the sinus node) controlling the atria and the other the ventricles. The ventricles may be controlled either from a junctional or ventricular focus. When these two pacemakers become further out of synchronization, the impulse from the atria may descend into the atrioventricular junction before the pacemaker from this area is ready to discharge again and the atrium then 'captures' the ventricles. There is, therefore, no organic block but only a physiological block due to the two pacemakers competing with each other. A-V dissociation is always secondary to some other abnormality, with either slowing of the sinus node or acceleration of a lower pacemaker, or a combination of the two.

Causes include:

Acute myocardial infarction
Digitalis toxicity

Treatment. No specific treatment is required although atropine sulphate or atrial pacing may be required for associated sinus bradycardia.

ECG. P waves 'march through' the QRS complexes (i.e. they are dissociated).
At some time the P waves are followed by a QRS at the normal interval (capture beats).

BUNDLE BRANCH BLOCK

In this condition either the right or the left branch of the A-V bundle fails to conduct impulses. Our understanding of bundle branch block has been greatly advanced by the development of A-V (His) bundle electrocardiographic recording. Bundle branch block often appears as a complication of ventricular hypertrophy, however a local lesion of the conducting system may be responsible for this condition.

The pathological significance of the two types of bundle branch block differs significantly. Right bundle branch block generally carries a good outlook. The prognosis of left bundle branch block is correspondingly more serious, because of the anatomical differences between this and the right bundle branch.

Right bundle branch block

In this condition there is a defect of conduction of the right bundle which gives rise to a characteristic electrocardiographic appearance as described earlier (in: abnormalities of the QRS complex). It is often an isolated congenital lesion of no importance, but may be associated with other congenital heart defects (particularly atrial septal defect). It occurs in acute pulmonary embolism, ischaemic heart disease, and right ventricular hypertrophy. Right bundle branch block may be partial (QRS width of less than 0.12 s) or complete (QRS is of 0.12 s duration or more). It is of little clinical significance, except as an indication of possible heart disease, and as a precursor of complete heart block.

Left bundle branch block

This condition is rare in the otherwise normal individual and is most commonly seen in ischaemic heart disease. It may also be seen in individuals with hypertension.

Neither form of bundle branch block requires treatment. The relatively new concepts of left anterior and left posterior hemiblock, and with them the terms single, bifasicular, and trifasicular block, are not discussed in detail here.

Hemiblocks

This is the term for blockage of one of the two main divisions of the left bundle branch (anterior and posterior). (*Rosenbaum et al 1970*)

Left anterior hemi-block. This condition is due to blockage of the anterior division of the left bundle branch. The spread of activation of the ventricle is consequently altered, producing left axis deviation (usually -60°).

Left posterior hemi-block. This rare condition is due to blockage of the posterior division of the left bundle branch. The altered spread of activation results in right axis deviation (usually +120°).

Right bundle branch with left anterior hemi-block. This is indicated by the combination of the right bundle branch block pattern in VI together with left axis deviation (usually –60°). Complete A-V block inevitably follows if the left posterior division becomes involved.

Right bundle branch with left posterior hemi-block. This is indicated by the unusual combination of the right bundle branch block pattern in VI together with right axis deviation (usually +120°). Complete A-V block follows if the anterior division of the left branch becomes diseased as well.

PRE-EXCITATION (WOLFF-PARKINSON-WHITE SYNDROME)

Accessory atrioventricular connexions are any muscle bundles which connect atrial and ventricular myocardium outside the junctional area. The accessory connexion which produces Wolff - Parkinson - White

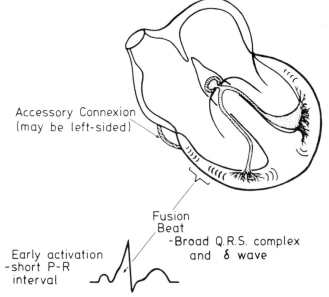

Fig. 49. *Diagrammatic representation of Wolff-Parkinson-White syndrome.*

(WPW) syndrome results in the characteristic electrocardiographic appearance of a shortened P-R internal (less than 0.11 s) associated with a prolonged QRS complex, the first upstroke of which is an abnormal slurred (delta) wave. (*Wolff et al 1930*)

This syndrome is associated with a liability to paroxysmal supraventricular tachycardia (SVT). The occurrence of SVT is attributable to the normal and abnormal conduction pathways forming a re-entry circuit.

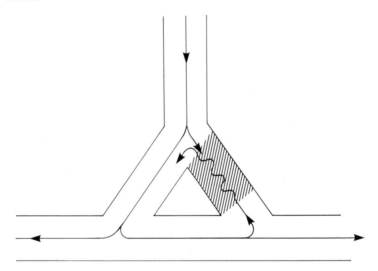

Fig. 50. *Diagram showing one of the forms of re-entrant re-excitation.*

WPW syndrome has been divided into two groups, A and B. Group A have predominantly positive ventricular complexes in VI, whereas group B complexes in VI are predominantly negative. (*Schamroth 1981*)

SICK SINUS SYNDROME (SINOATRIAL DISORDER)

This is a condition that occurs transiently in acute myocardial infarction. It is sometimes referred to as the *tachycardia–bradycardia syndrome*, in which bursts of an atrial tachyarrhythmia, usually atrial fibrillation, alternate with prolonged periods of sinus bradycardia. Where the ventricular rate is very fast, syncope may occur during the tachycardia.

Sick sinus syndrome was considered a rarity at one time, now it is one of the commonest conditions considered for pacing. A pacemaker is usually considered as treatment of choice, because drug therapy is usually disappointing. Only a small proportion of cases respond to atropine or isoprenaline.

FUSION BEATS

These are beats resulting from the simultaneous spread of more than one impulse through the same area of the myocardium (either ventricles or atria). Fusion beats, also known as *summation* or *combination* beats, are seen when ectopic beats occur late in diastole, and in parasystole when the parasystolic impulse happens to coincide with a sinus beat. They are also commonly seen in accelerated idioventricular rhythms and when the heart is being artificially paced. Fusion beats interrupting tachycardia are often called Dressler beats.

Fusion beats can be recognized on the ECG by the QRS complex having a configuration intermediate between the two beats (often the 'pure' sinus beat, and the 'pure' ventricular beat.

PARASYSTOLE

Parasystole is an independent, ectopic rhythm that operates alongside the primary rhythm, and whose pacemaker is 'protected' from outside impulses. Because the ectopic pacemaking centre is 'protected' (the physiological hallmark of parasystole) it is able to maintain its rhythm without interruption. (*Schamroth 1981*)

In parasystole both pacemakers activate the same area of myocardium. The parasystolic centre is usually ventricular.

Parasystole can be recognized on the EEG by a variation in coupling intervals and by a common denominator in the interectopic intervals.

ABERRANT CONDUCTION

Aberrant ventricular conduction (ventricular aberration) is the temporary, abnormal intraventricular conduction (bundle branch block) of supraventricular impulses.

Its importance lies in the ability to distinguish it from ventricular arrhythmias for which it is frequently misdiagnosed. More commonly it can be recognized by a bizarre QRS complex resembling a right bundle branch block pattern.

Interpolation

An interpolated ventricular ectopic beat is an ectopic beat which is 'sandwiched' between two conducted sinus beats. It therefore occurs without a compensatory pause. Interpolated ectopic beats are usually associated with slow sinus rhythms.

REFERENCES

Barold, S.S. & Coumol, P. (1977) Mechanisms of atrioventricular junctional tachycardia: role of re-entry and concealed accessory by-pass tracts. *Am. J. Cardiol.*, *39*, 97.

Einthoven, W. (1903). Die galvanometrische Registrierung des menschlichen Elecktrokardiogramme: Zugleich eine Beurteilung der Anwendung des Capillar-elecktrometers in der Physiologie. *Pfugers Archiv fur die gesarnbe Physiologie des Menschen und der Tiere*, *99*, 472.

Hollifield, J.W. & Statton, P.E. (1980) Thiazide diuretics, hypokalaemia and cardiac arrhythmias. *Acta med. Scand.*, *647* (Suppl.), 67.

Olsson, S.B. (1980) Nature of cardiac arrhythmias and electrolyte disturbances: role of potassium in A.F. *Acta med. Scand.*, *647*, 83.

Pilcher, J. & Nagle, R.E. (1971) Acid-base imbalance and arrhythmias after myocardial infarction. *Br. Heart J.*, *33*, 526.

Rosenbaum, M.B., Elizari, M.V. & Lazzari, J.O. (1970) *The hemiblocks*. Tampa tracings, Oldsmar, Florida.

Schamroth, L. (1981) *The electrocardiology of coronary artery disease*. Oxford: Blackwell Scientific Publications.

Seller, R.H., Cangiano, J., Kim, K.E., Mendelssohn, S., Brest, A.N. & Swartz, C. (1970) Digitalis toxicity and hypomagnesemia. *Am. Heart J.*, *79*, 57.

Shaw, D.B. & Kekasick, C.A. (1978) Potential candidates for pacemakers, surveys of heart block and sino-atrial disorder (sick-sinus-syndrome). *Br. Heart J.*, *40*, 99.

Spurrell, R.A.J. & Camm, A.J. (1978) Surgical treatment of ventricular tachycardia. *Br. Heart J.*, *40*, 38 (Suppl.).

Thompson, D.R. (1979) An introduction to cardiac arrhythmias. *Nurs. Mirror 149*, 19 (Suppl.).

Wolff, L., Parkinson, J. & White, P.D. (1930) Bundle-branch block with short PR interval in healthy young people prone to paroxysmal tachycardia. *Am. Heart J.*, *5*, 685.

4
Heart Disease

METHODS OF CARDIAC EXAMINATION

The techniques of inspection, palpation and auscultation are generally more helpful than percussion in determining the cardiac status of the individual.

INSPECTION

This should include observation of the body build, skin, chest symmetry, neck vein pulsations, precordial (chest) movement, and the extremities. The apical impulse, which is caused by the contraction of the left ventricle, may be visible in about 50% of normal adults in the mid-left clavicular line at the 5th interspace.

PALPATION

Information gathered from inspection is augmented using the technique of palpation. Palpation consists of a systemic examination of the chest. The location, size and character of the apical impulse should be identified. *Thrills* are palpable murmurs caused by abnormal blood flow and may be observed as a sort of purring sensation. Palpation with the palmar aspect of the base of the fingers best picks up vibrations, while palpation with the fingertips best discloses pulsations.

PERCUSSION

This is less helpful in determining cardiac status than other techniques of examination. Formerly, percussion was used to determine heart size. However, it is of no value for this nowadays. Dullness in the second intercostal space suggests the possibility of an aneurysm of the aorta or enlargement of the pulmonary artery.

AUSCULTATION

Auscultation of the heart sounds is performed first with the patient in a supine position. The auscultatory sites are the points on the chest to which the sounds are best transmitted, not the anatomical location of the valves. The *first heart sound* (S_1) is created by vibrations from the closing of the mitral and tricuspid valves. The *second heart sound* (S_2) represents the closing of the aortic and pulmonary valves. Using the diaphragm of the stethoscope and starting at the second right intercostal space, one can hear these heart sounds. S_1 may be louder at the apex, while S_2 may be louder at the base of the heart.

During inspiration, there may be normal physiological splitting of the second heart sound into two components, A_2 and P_2. This is caused by increased venous return to the right side of the heart during inspiration and by a prolonged delay in the closing of the pulmonary valve. Physiological splitting may not be audible in some individuals.

A *third heart sound* (ventricular gallop) occurs after S_2, and is produced by vibrations of the ventricles due to rapid distension. A *fourth heart sound* (atrial gallop) occurs in late diastole and is thought to result from vibrations of the valves, supporting structures, or ventricles during the atrial systolic ejection of blood into the ventricles.

An *ejection click* caused by stenosis of the aortic or pulmonary valve may be heard. Another abnormal heart sound is an *opening snap of the mitral valve* associated with a thickened mitral valve.

HEART MURMURS

Murmurs may be caused by:

1. Increased flow through normal structures.
2. Forward flow across a stenotic valve.
3. Backward flow through an incompetent valve.

4. Flow from a high pressure chamber or vessel through an abnormal passage.
5. Flow into a dilated chamber.

Murmurs are evaluated according to their timing, location, intensity, pitch, quality and radiation. The timing of a murmur may be systolic or diastolic, and it may be present in all or part of the cardiac cycle. Murmurs heard throughout systole are called *holosystolic* or *pansystolic*. They may be of equal intensity throughout or may exhibit a crescendo-decrescendo pattern. The intensity is graded on a scale of 1 – 6, with 1 being very faint and 6 being audible even when the stethoscope is slightly raised from the chest. Pitch may be high, medium or low. The quality may be harsh, blowing, rumbling or musical. Locations of murmurs are described according to the intercostal position and the distance from the midsternal, midclavicular, or one of the axillary lines.

ARTERIAL PULSES

The radial pulse is convenient and the conventional site for examination, but the larger carotid or femoral pulse is better for assessment of tension and quality. An examination of arterial pulses should include palpating all the major pulses individually, and then comparing the pulse of one side of the body with the corresponding pulse on the other. If an irregular pulse is noted, one should also observe whether there is correlation with the respiratory cycle. The pulse should be counted for one minute and then compared with the apical rate for a minute. If the apical rate exceeds the peripheral rate, a *peripheral pulse deficit* is said to exist. When the arterial pulse is examined, the following characteristics should be noted: *rate, rhythm, amplitude (tension)* and *quality* or *wave form*.

The rate of the pulse in the normal resting adult averages 70 per minute. In the newborn infant the rate is 140 per minute, and in a child of eight years it has decreased to 90 per minute. An increased rate *(tachycardia)* is usually due to nervousness. Other causes of simple sinus tachycardia are fever, thyrotoxicosis, anaemia, and drugs including alcohol and tobacco. Exercise also causes rates in excess of 100 per minute. A slow rate *(bradycardia)* as low as 40 per minute may be found in the healthy and particularly the athletic. However it may be indicative of heart block.

The normal pulse is regular or exhibits sinus arrhythmia. Ectopic beats (extrasystoles) may be present. A coupling of beats (*pulsus bigeminus*) is due to the alternation of normal and ectopic beats. A totally irregular pulse suggests atrial fibrillation.

The amplitude of the pulse depends on the *pulse pressure* (the difference between the systolic and diastolic pressures). The pulse is of small volume when the pulse pressure is small. Pulses of large volume are produced by large stroke volumes.

Types of pulse

Anacrotic pulse. A slow upstroke associated with a pulse wave of low amplitude. A notch is felt on the upstroke. Occurs in aortic stenosis.

Pulsus bisferiens. A notch at the peak of a pulse wave of large volume. A double beat can be felt. Occurs in aortic stenosis with regurgitation.

Pulsus alternans. Evenly spaced alternate stronger and weaker beats. Occurs in left ventricular failure.

Pulsus paradoxus. The pulse volume becomes much smaller during inspiration and larger during expiration. Occurs in asthma and tamponade.

Collapsing pulse. A large volume pulse which rises rapidly and collapses suddenly. This 'water-hammer' (Corrigan's) pulse may be seen in the carotid arteries. Occurs in aortic incompetence and in persistent ductus arteriosus (PDA).

BLOOD PRESSURE

The intermittent rise and fall of pressure within the arteries depends on the ejection of blood from the left ventricle. The peak pressure is called the *systolic pressure* and the lowest pressure the *diastolic pressure*. The difference between systolic and diastolic pressure is called the *pulse pressure*.

Blood pressure depends on the cardiac output and the peripheral resistance to blood flow. An increase in cardiac output causes a rise in mean blood pressure, the systolic pressure being more affected than the diastolic pressure. A rise in resistance to flow causes a rise in mean blood pressure. The rise in blood pressure which occurs on exercise or with emotion is predominantly due to a rise in cardiac output and this may often be associated with a fall in peripheral resistance. Elasticity of the arteries is another factor which modifies the blood pressure. With increasing age the arteries become less elastic and the pulse pressure increases.

When measuring the blood pressure the patient must be resting, comfortable and composed. The blood pressure varies throughout the day, falling to low levels during sleep and rising to high levels with anxiety or exercise. Isolated blood pressure recordings can therefore prove misleading. Blood pressure varies according to age. In an infant levels of 100/60 mmHg would be normal; in the 20 year old, blood pressure taken at rest varies between 100/60 – 140/90 mmHg. There is a tendency for average blood pressure to rise smoothly and steadily with advancing years. This affects particularly the systolic pressure. (*Thompson 1981*)

Circadian blood pressure change

Over a 24 hour period, wide fluctuations in blood pressure are observed. The lowest pressures are recorded during sleep. It falls to a minimum during the first hour of sleep, remains low for several hours, rising between 0500 – 0700 hours. During the waking hours, spikes of blood pressure elevation occur with physical and mental stress.

BLOOD PRESSURE RECORDING

It is well documented that there are many sources of error in recording blood pressure, including poor technique and observer bias. The nurse must be able to carry out this important procedure with care and accuracy. The sphygmomanometer is the commonest and most important measuring instrument used by the nurse, and yet its use is the least subject to any kind of quality control. Nurses frequently record blood pressure and the measurements they obtain affect decisions on treatment, investigations, and prognosis. When the nurse measures blood pressure routinely, the reading is assumed to be accurate. Many nurses are unaware of potential errors of technique and fail to appreciate the limits of the measurement.

Adequate explanation of the procedure is important to allay the fears of the anxious patient. The patient should avoid exertion and not eat or smoke for thirty minutes beforehand. The room should be comfortable, warm and quiet, and the patient should be allowed to rest for at least five minutes before the measurement.

The arm should be unclothed and supported, otherwise the patient will perform isometric exercises which may give false readings. The nurse should also be in a comfortable relaxed position. If she is hurried she will release the pressure too rapidly thus giving false readings. The nurse should wrap the cuff round the patient's arm, ensuring that the bladder dimensions are accurate (20% greater than the diameter of the limb to be measured). The brachial artery is palpated with one hand, and the cuff rapidly inflated to about 30 mmHg above the disappearance of the pulse and then slowly deflated. The nurse should note the pressure at which the pulse reappears. This is the approximate level of the systolic pressure. The stethoscope should be applied to the antecubital fossa over the brachial artery. A bell endpiece gives better sound reproduction, but a diaphragm is easier to secure with the fingers of one hand. The stethoscope should be applied firmly, but with the minimum amount of pressure. The stethoscope should not be touching clothing or the cuff. With the stethoscope in place, the cuff is inflated rapidly to about 30 mmHg above the palpated systolic pressure and deflated at a rate of 2 mmHg/s. As the pressure falls the Korotkoff sounds become audible. The appearance of sounds (phase I) should be recorded as the systolic pressure. The disappearance of sounds (phase 5) should be recorded as the diastolic pressure. However, some people prefer to record phase 4 (muffling of sounds) as the diastolic pressure. Whichever is used should be predetermined, and recorded in writing. The pressures should be recorded to the nearest 2 mmHg. When all sounds have disappeared, the cuff should be deflated rapidly and completely. One or two minutes should elapse before further measurements are made. (*Thompson 1981*)

The blood pressure should be measured on at least two separate occasions. If the blood pressure is increased, the mean recording should be noted.

The method of blood pressure measurement outlined above is the indirect method. A more accurate direct method involves the insertion of a miniaturized pressure transducer unit into an artery for the transmission of a wave form or digital display on a monitor. (*Raferty 1978*)

The patient's blood pressure should be recorded in both arms. A difference of 5 mmHg is not uncommon, and the arm with the highest recording, should be subsequently used for measurements. Whatever positions are used, they should be specified with the following abbreviations: L (lying) or S (standing); RA (right arm) or LA (left arm); the presence of any arrhythmias, anxiety or confinement to bed should also be recorded.

CENTRAL VENOUS PRESSURE

As mentioned earlier, distension of the jugular vein may indicate elevated venous pressure and subsequent heart failure. The normal central venous pressure (CVP), the pressure in the right atrium or the superior vena cava, is about 3 – 10 cm H_2O. Measurements of CVP are not infrequent in acute cardiac areas, and the procedure involves a good deal of nursing expertise. A measuring catheter is inserted into the superior vena cava via a vein in the antecubital fossa. Less commonly the subclavian or internal jugular vein are catheterized. From this catheter, the pressure can be measured by using a manometer, a three-way tap, and the infusion bottle, which may contain dextrose, dextrose saline or normal saline.

When a measurement is to be taken, the patient should preferably (if able) lie flat in bed, and the O reading on the manometer should be level with the right atrium. Reference points may be the sternal angle or the mid-axillary line. A spirit level is used to ascertain this. The tap is then turned so that the fluid fills the manometer. The tap is then turned so that the fluid goes from the manometer to the patient. When the fluid level in the manometer remains relatively stable (but respiratory oscillations are present), it is equal to the pressure in the venous system. At this point the measurement (CVP) is read. It is important to turn the tap to the position that allows fluid to flow from the infusion bottle to the patient. The infusion rate is usually kept low just to keep the vein and catheter patent.

The measurement is usually made every two hours, or much more frequently, depending on the circumstances. It is an important indication of the patient's circulatory and cardiac state. (*Holland 1977*)

JUGULAR VENOUS PRESSURE AND PULSE

Examination of the jugular venous pulse and pressure assesses the function of the right heart.

Jugular venous pulsations consist of several components, owing to various physiological events in the cardiac cycle. These components can be seen as a diffuse undulating movement and are not palpable. Both the internal and external jugular veins may be examined, but the internal jugular is a more reliable indicator.

Full neck veins may be visible in an individual with normal venous pressure in the supine position. When the patient is lying at an angle of $45°$, the jugular vein may be barely visible above the clavicles. However, if the venous pressure is elevated, the jugular veins may be visible all the way up to the angle of the jaw when the patient is in an upright position. Venous pressure is measured by observing the number of centimetres above the sternal angle that venous pulses can be seen. The sternal angle is a relatively constant distance of 5 – 7 cm above the right atrium.

The most common cause of raised jugular venous pressure is right ventricular failure secondary to left heart failure. Increased blood volume and increased pressure within the pericardium are other possible causes.

The components of the jugular venous pulsations are normally three positive waves, a, c, and v, and two negative waves, x and y. The 'a' wave is produced by a rise of pressure due to atrial systole. The negative 'x' wave is produced by the fall of pressure caused by atrial relaxation. The 'c' wave is a carotid artefact, and is not usually possible to see in the jugular pulse. Blood continues to flow into the atrium during atrial relaxation, causing a rise in atrial pressure which produces the positive 'v' wave. When the tricuspid valve opens in early diastole the atrial pressure falls producing the negative 'y' wave.

Cannon waves

If the atrium contracts when the tricuspid valve is closed (as in ventricular systole), a jet of blood is forced into the jugular veins and a visible 'cannon' wave results. They occur intermittently in complete heart block and in ventricular tachycardia when atrial and ventricular systoles coincide. In nodal (junctional) rhythms, atrial and ventricular contractions are synchronous and cannon waves are therefore regular with every heart beat.

TECHNIQUES OF INVESTIGATION

RADIOLOGY

Radiological investigation of the heart and pulmonary circulation is an invaluable part of the full cardiological assessment. These interpretations are related to clinical, electrocardiographic and other findings.

X-rays, because of their short wave length can penetrate materials which do not transmit visible light. They were discovered by Conrad Röentgen (1895) who was then an obscure German physicist.

Simple X-ray

A great deal can be learned from a careful study of the cardiac contours and of the lung fields as shown in a simple postero-anterior (P-A) film of the chest. X-rays detect heart shape, lung vessel changes and interstitial oedema. These may demonstrate various conditions, e.g. mitral stenosis, cardiac enlargement, coarctation of the aorta, etc.

Screening (Fluoroscopy)

Observation of the heart on the image intensifier is of some value in assessing selective chamber enlargement. A barium swallow may also be helpful, since the barium-filled oesophagus is displaced in a typical manner by the enlarged left atrium of mitral stenosis.

CARDIAC CATHETERIZATION AND ANGIOGRAPHY

Introduction

Cardiac catheterization can be defined as the insertion into one or more

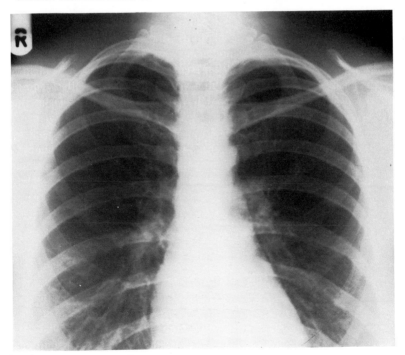

Fig. 51. *X-ray of a normal heart.*

of the heart chambers (usually under screening) of a fine flexible catheter. The procedure is performed under sterile conditions in a cardiac laboratory equipped with facilities for screening, cine-filming, and video-tape recording; multi-channel pressure recording; blood gas estimation; anaesthesia; and resuscitation. (*Mendel 1974*)

The right and left hearts may be investigated separately or together. Cardiac catheterization is mainly performed to:

1. Visualize the heart chambers and vessels by means of radiopaque substances under X-ray control.
2. Measure pressures and record the wave forms from the cavity of the heart chambers and great vessels.
3. Obtain blood samples from the heart for the measurement of cardiac output and the identification of intracardiac shunts.

Right heart catheterization
A catheter is introduced into the right atrium via a basilic or saphenous vein. The catheter is usually passed over a guide wire which has been introduced into the vein through a cannula; this is known as the Seldinger technique. Once the catheter enters the right atrium it is manoeuvred through the tricuspid valve to the ventricle, then to the pulmonary artery, and is eventually wedged in a distal pulmonary artery, where the pulmonary arterial wedge pressure is obtained. Sampling and pressures are obtained on the gradual withdrawal of the catheter. The pulmonary arterial wedge pressure is used as a record of indirect left atrial pressure. (*Swan et al 1970*)

Right heart catheterization is useful for diagnosing forms of congenital and some acquired heart disease, e.g. pulmonary hypertension, pulmonary valvar stenosis, and atrial septal defect and ventricular septal defect.

Left heart catheterization
When more specific information than the left atrial pressure is required, then the left heart needs to be entered. Several techniques are employed:

Retrograde aortic technique. A catheter is introduced into the brachial or femoral artery and is advanced into the aorta, through the aortic valve and into the left ventricle. (*Jodkins 1967*)

Trans-septal technique. A catheter is introduced into the *right* atrium using a stilette as a guide. The trans-septal needle carefully perforates the interatrial septum. The catheter is then passed over the needle into the left atrium and the needle itself withdrawn. The catheter may then be advanced into the left ventricle. (*Rushkind and Miller 1966*)

Direct left ventricle needle puncture. A catheter is introduced into the left ventricle by means of a puncture through the chest wall. This technique is practically obsolete now.

Left heart catheterization is useful for recording pressures, estimating oxygen saturation of extracted blood samples, and for allowing angiocardiography. It is also used for diagnosing aortic valve stenosis.

OTHER RESULTS OBTAINABLE

If the oxygen content of the blood in the pulmonary artery and brachial artery and the oxygen consumption are known, the cardiac output can be calculated from the Fick formula:

$$\text{Cardiac output (litre/min)} = \frac{\text{Oxygen consumption (ml/min)}}{\text{Arterio-venous oxygen difference (ml/litre)}}$$

The area of a valve can be calculated if the pressure difference across it, and the forward flow throughout are known. Similarly, the volume of a shunt can be calculated from the measurement of relevant oxygen saturation in conjunction with oxygen uptake.

The angiocardiogram can be performed for estimation of left ventricular size and function. Evidence of mitral incompetence and the site of any obstruction can be demonstrated.

ANGIOCARDIOGRAPHY

A radiopaque contrast medium is quickly injected into the heart or great vessels. Rapid successive X-ray films are then taken. These high-speed cine-films are taken at about 80–200 frames per second, and can be played back immediately, by the use of video recording.

Complications are uncommon, but of importance nonetheless. Perforation of the heart or a great vessel, syncope, transient cardiac arrhythmias including ventricular ectopic beats, atrial ectopic beats, asystole and ventricular fibrillation (uncommon) and varying degrees of heart block may occur.

APEXCARDIOGRAPHY

An apexcardiogram (ACG) is the recording of the movement of the cardiac apex as a simple displacement curve, and provides a record of the sensation which can be felt with the hand when the apex beat is palpated.

It is of value as a very useful reference point in phonocardiography. It provides possible detection of early left ventricular stress in diseases such as systemic hypertension, aortic stenosis and ischaemic heart disease. It is also of value in detecting mitral stenosis.

THERMOGRAPHY

In thermography the variations in the amount of heat constantly being emitted by infra-red radiation from the body structures are detected and recorded so as to produce a visual image. The method is a simple and quite harmless technique.

In cardiology, its uses are limited to the investigation of arterial disease, where it can be used to evaluate narrowing or obstruction of the carotid vessels.

COMPUTED TOMOGRAPHY

Computerised transverse axial tomography (CT scanning) is a new non-invasive method of body imaging in which a digital computer is employed to analyze radiographic data. As in all tomography, the image produced is that of a 'slice' of tissue — usually 0.8 mm – 1.5 mm thick. This remarkably accurate diagnostic technique was introduced in the UK by G.N. Hounsfield in 1972, and developed by EMI. It was first used clinically at the Atkinson-Morleys Hospital in London. It is said to be the most important advance in radiology since the discovery of X-rays. It differs from conventional X-ray systems in that X-ray film is replaced by a system of crystal detectors and a computer. The various tissues within the body absorb radiation differently, and are ultimately represented by various colours in a picture reconstructed by the computer. Each colour represents a certain radiation absorption factor.

Originally the use of this technique was confined to the investigations of the brain. In cardiology its uses are limited at present. It can be used to diagnose pericardial and pleural effusions and mediastinal masses.

NUCLEAR IMAGING

This is a relatively new technique which can be used to investigate the heart using radioisotopes and gamma cameras with computer processing facilities. These isotopes (e.g. Thallium 201 and Potassium 43) can be injected which are taken up by cardiac lesions. These increased local concentrations of radioisotopes are detected by a scintillator crystal which is linked to photo-multipliers and a recorder. This technique is used for the measurement of total coronary flow, systolic and diastolic volumes of the heart. It is useful in detecting pericardial effusions and shunts. Several congenital cardiac anomalies including single ventricle, Fallots tetralogy and pulmonary atresia can be diagnosed by these methods. (*Rowlands et al 1981*)

ECHOCARDIOGRAPHY

Echocardiography, another non-invasive technique employes pulses of high-frequency sound waves (ultrasound) emitted from a transducer to evaluate patients with valvular heart disease, congenital heart disease, cardiomyopathy, ischaemic heart disease or pericardial disease. The ultrasonic waves in echocardiography have a frequency range of millions of cycles per second. Ultrasound will travel in straight lines unless it is reflected or refracted by an interface between two different structures or tissues. More sound waves will be reflected if the ultrasonic beam is directly perpendicular to the plane of a structure. Various areas within the heart may be identified by their characteristic patterns of motion. (*Donaldson 1981*)

In recording an echocardiogram, the transducer is placed in the fourth intercostal space at the left sternal border and is aimed in various directions to visualize cardiac and valvular motion. As the ultrasonic beam passes through the cardiac structures, echoes are reflected to the transducer, which converts them into electricity. The resulting wave patterns are then displayed on an oscilloscope and can be recorded on film.

Echocardiography is helpful in detecting abnormalities such as mitral stenosis and incompetence, vegetation and calcification of the mitral valve, aortic stenosis and incompetence, tricuspid valve disease, left ventricular function and pericardial effusion.

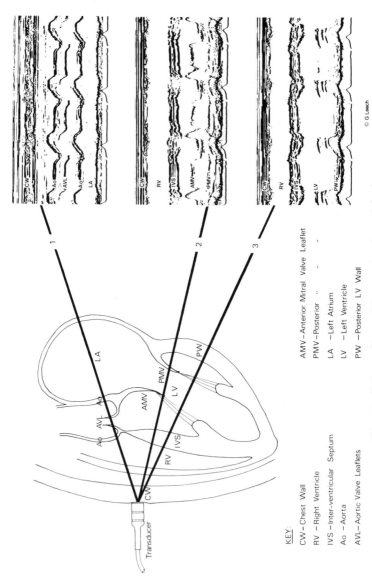

Fig. 52. *Echocardiographic examination of the heart.*

KEY:

CW – Chest Wall

RV – Right Ventricle

IVS – Inter-ventricular Septum

Ao – Aorta

AVL – Aortic Valve Leaflets

AMV – Anterior Mitral Valve Leaflet

PMV – Posterior " " "

LA – Left Atrium

LV – Left Ventricle

PW – Posterior LV Wall

PHONOCARDIOGRAPHY

Phonocardiography is a means of graphically recording the sounds made during various events in the cardiac cycle. This non-invasive procedure identifies normal heart sounds, murmurs, gallops, opening snaps, ejection sounds and clicks. The amplitude of the waves in phonocardiography is a measure of the intensity of the sounds; it corresponds with grading the murmurs, from grade I – VI on auscultation. The number of waves per unit of time is the frequency. Low frequency murmurs are seen in patients with aortic or pulmonary stenosis. The timing of sounds in relationship to physiological events can be achieved by simultaneously recording the electrocardiogram, apexcardiogram, or carotid pulse. (*Leatham 1979*)

The phonocardiogram (PCG) is *not* of value in routine clinical practice.

REMOTE (TAPE) MONITORING ELECTROCARDIOGRAPHY

These monitoring techniques provide practical methods of taking continuous long-duration (usually 24 hours or more), single- or two-lead ECGs. This method is now established as an invaluable aid in the documentation of arrhythmias (symptomatic and asymptomatic) which occur in ordinary life as well as in hospital. (*Harrison et al 1978*)

There are several different systems available, all consisting of two basic units.

Tape-recorder

A small, battery operated transistorized tape-recorder which can be carried in a shoulder-strap at the side.

Scanner

A scanner which permits the display and analysis of the tape recording in a variety of ways and in a very much shorter period than if the tape were to be played back beat by beat in 'real-time'.

INTRA-CARDIAC RECORDING

Various techniques of intra-cardiac recording are used to study arrhythmias. His bundle electrocardiography (HBE) is of particular interest and has enhanced our understanding of arrhythmias, especially atrioventricular block.

This system consists of electrodes for recording and stimulation, recording equipment, circuit and stimulator.

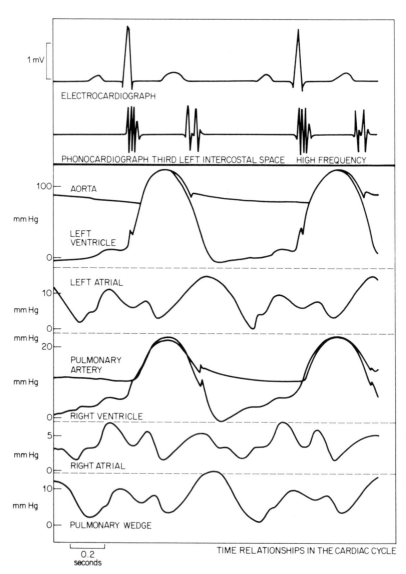

Fig. 53. *Time relationships in the cardiac cycle.*

Computer application to ECGs

Many CCUs now have a computer programme which provides continuous analysis of the ECG and an immediate alert of rhythm change. In addition, the computer can examine more ECG data, store, retrieve, correlate, and statistically manipulate it.

The computer measurement of amplitudes, duration, and intervals is extremely accurate. Unfortunately, ECG standardization does not properly exist, and therefore ECG interpretation is a highly individualistic exercise.

Computers in haemodynamic monitoring

The computer is often used to make recordings of left ventricular function from pulmonary artery pressure (PAP), left ventricular pressure (LVP), and cardiac output (CO) as measured by the thermodilution method. A computer that calculates cardiac index and body surface area is also now available.

EXERCISE (STRESS) TESTING

Indications

1. Evaluation of functional capacity.
2. 'Diagnosis' of IHD (see Chapter 7, p. 142).
3. Detection of cardiac arrhythmias.
4. Assessment of response to treatment:
   Drugs
   Surgery
   Rehabilitation
5. Screening of special groups:
   Pilots
   PSV and HGV licence holders
   Intending joggers
6. Prediction of prognosis.

Contra-indications

There are no absolute contra-indications to exercise testing, but care should be taken in patients with recent infarction, unstable angina, heart failure, arrhythmias at rest, severe valve disease (aortic stenosis), or recent viral infection.

A resting ECG should be taken before beginning exercise. The blood pressure should be recorded before, during, and after the test.

ST segment changes

The criteria for ischaemic ST segments are still not agreed upon. Unfortunately, certain known factors, including potassium and digitalis, affect ST segment morphology, therefore ST segment depression is not specific for ischaemia (i.e., false positive responses may occur). It is, however, generally agreed that ST segment depression denotes an increased degree of ischaemia.

A positive exercise test is one which shows horizontal depression of the ST segment 0.5 mm (0.05 mV) or more below the base-line. Interpretation is often difficult and many patients with obvious angina do not have a positive ECG exercise test.

Precautions

Exercise testing should be done in a setting where emergencies can be dealt with quickly and efficiently. An emergency supply of appropriate drugs should be readily available, together with syringes, IV equipment, ambu-bag and oxygen. A DC defibrillator should also be on hand although it will be rarely used.

IMPLICATIONS FOR THE NURSE

The responsibility of the nurse in diagnostic tests varies greatly according to the nature of the test and the particular situation. In many cases they are responsible for the preparation of the patients, the equipment to be used, and the collection of specimens. However, more importantly, they are responsible for the safety and comfort of the patient, for example, after arterial puncture.

Patients are interested in the diagnostic tests in a number of ways, i.e.; why and how the test is carried out, on what part of the body it is made, what they can do to help with the test, what the results of the test will indicate, when they will be told the results, and if the person performing the test is competent. They will also want to know if more tests are going to be necessary. The nurse can help by giving preparatory information (i.e. the sensations they might expect to experience during the procedure), which is more effective than simply describing the actual procedure.

REFERENCES

Donaldson, R. Sounding out the heart. *Nurs. Mirror*, *152* (15), 40.

Harrison, D.C., Fitzgerald, S.W. & Winkle, R.A. (1978) Contribution of ambulatory electrocardiographic monitoring to antiarrhythmic management. *Am. J. Cardiol.*, *41*, 996.

Holland, (1977) *Cardiovascular nursing: prevention, intervention and rehabilitation.* Boston: Little, Brown & Co.

Judkins, M.P. (1967) Selective coronary arteriography. A percutaneous transfemoral technique. *Radiology*, *89*, 815.

Leatham, A. (1979). *Auscultation of the heart and phonocardiography.* Edinburgh: Churchill Livingstone.

Mendel, D. (1974) *A practice of cardiac catheterization.* Oxford: Blackwell Scientific Publications.

Raftery, E.B. (1978) The methodology of blood pressure recording. *Br. J. clin. Pharmacol.*, *6*, 193.

Roëntgen, C. (1895) *Eine neve Art von Strahlen.* In: *A short history of medicine* (1962) ed. C. Singer & E.A. Underwood. Oxford: Clarendon Press.

Rowlands, D.J., Shields, R.A. & Testa, H.J. (1981) *Radionucleides in cardiology.* In: *Recent advances in cardiology* (ed. J. Homes & D.J. Rowlands) Edinburgh: Churchill Livingstone.

Rushkind, W.J. & Miller, W.W. (1966) Creation of an A.S.D. without thoracotomy. *J. Am. med. Assoc.*, *196*, 991.

Swan, H.J.C., Ganz, W., Forrester, J., Marcus, H., Diamond, G. & Chonette, D. (1970) Catheterization of the heart in man with use of a flow-directed balloon tipped catheter. *New Engl. J. Med.*, *283*, 447.

Thompson, D.R. (1981) Recording patients' blood pressure: a review. *J. adv. Nurs.*, *6*, 283.

5
General Principles
of Patient Care

BASIC NURSING CONCEPTS

Before going on to discuss the unique role of the nurse in caring for the individual with heart disease, it is pertinent to outline some basic nursing concepts. This includes:

The role of the nurse
Activities of living
Models of living
Health care systems
Process of nursing

THE ROLE OF THE NURSE

There have been many attempts at defining the role of the nurse and none is universally acceptable. Virginia Henderson's is probably that which has been most widely accepted as a basis for discussion.

'The unique function of the nurse is to assist the individual, sick and well, in the performance of those activities contributing to health or its recovery (or to a peaceful death) that he would perform unaided if he had the necessary strength, will or knowledge. And to do this in such a way as to help him gain independence as rapidly as possible.' (*Henderson 1960*)

From this, some important facts can be abstracted:

1. Nursing consists essentially of acts of helping or assistance.
2. There is a nursing role in respect of well people as well as sick people (i.e. preventive role).
3. The major focus of nursing is on activities which people normally do for themselves (i.e. 'self-care activities' *or* 'activities of living').
4. The nursing role takes in physical and psychological assistance and it has a teaching function.

There is probably need for more conscious decision making about the amount of medically derived work undertaken by the nurse, and its repercussions on the unique role of the nurse. Tasks allocated by the doctor are often repetitive ones requiring relatively little skill. If too much emphasis is placed on these technical skills, the caring role of the nurse may be crowded out. The caring role is then delegated to the less skilled and ultimately standards of care deteriorate. (*McFarlane 1980*)

The nurse is the link between what are often stressful, complicated technical procedures associated with the disease process and the maintenance of everyday physical and psychological functions which are so important to the patient's comfort, and to him as an individual.

The process of nursing (Nursing Process) may be seen as a scientific framework for developing the nursing care which is relevant to the individual problems of the patient. It has several dynamics relevant to all the components of nursing in terms of nursing practice, theory, management, education and research. These must be foremost in all future nursing developments.

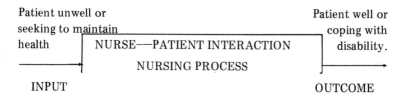

Patient unwell or seeking to maintain health

NURSE—PATIENT INTERACTION

NURSING PROCESS

Patient well or coping with disability.

INPUT

OUTCOME

ACTIVITIES OF LIVING

These are:

Maintaining a safe environment
Communicating
Breathing
Eating and drinking
Eliminating
Control of body temperature
Sleeping
Personal hygiene and dressing
Working
Playing
Expressing sexuality
Dying

(Roper et al 1981)
Although every activity of living (AL) is important, some are more vital than others. The AL of prime importance is breathing. ALs reflect human needs. Human needs can be categorized in order of priority creating a hierarchy of them:

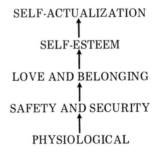

SELF-ACTUALIZATION

SELF-ESTEEM

LOVE AND BELONGING

SAFETY AND SECURITY

PHYSIOLOGICAL

Maslow's (1970) version of human needs is probably the best known to nurses, and is outlined here:

Physiological needs: those involved in maintaining bodily processes.
Safety and security needs: the need to avoid danger or anything that may harm the individual.
Belonging and love needs: the need to give love and affection by another person or persons.

Esteem needs: the need to be valued, accepted, and appreciated as a person; to achieve and be adequate; to acquire status, recognition and attention.

Self-actualization: the need for self-fulfilment.

According to Maslow, biological needs must be satisfied before an individual can turn his attention to higher needs. Although higher needs can be postponed and are less urgent, living at the level of higher needs leads to greater biological efficiency.

Nursing must meet all those needs which fall within its scope (within the resources available) and these may fall into any of Maslow's five categories.

MODELS OF LIVING

Life-span of living
Living is concerned with the whole of a person's life (*life-span*) from conception to death.

CONCEPTION ■——— LIFE-SPAN ———→ DEATH

Dependence/independence in living
There are certain periods in life when a person cannot yet, or can no longer, perform certain ALs. Each person could be said to have a dependent/independent continuum for each activity along which movement can take place in either direction. (*Roper et al 1980*)

TOTALLY ←——— CONTINUUM ———→ TOTALLY
DEPENDENT   INDEPENDENT

HEALTH CARE SYSTEMS

The usual method of providing care in use today has been thought of as a 'hospital-based' or 'medical-based' model of health care. For some time it has been under criticism because it has extended to only a small proportion of the general population.

It is now becoming obvious that a greater emphasis needs to be placed on delivering community-based health care. Health care professionals have now begun to direct their attention to the desirability of maintaining and promoting health rather than concentrating so much on the individual's relatively isolated episodes of illness which are often treated in hospital.

Data base

There is a need to collect records about patient care which most members of the health team can use, and which can form a data base for decision-making about individual care. Recently computers have been introduced in an attempt to improve standards of patient care.

Many health care systems incorporate the problem-orientated approach to the recording of patient data: problem orientated medical records (POMR). This has provided a change of focus in records away from the disease and towards the patient and his problems. This type of record can be used by nurses only, or by other members of the multidisciplinary health team.

The objectives in collecting information about the activities of living (ALs) is to discover:

1. Previous routines.
2. What the patient can, and cannot do for himself.
3. Problems and discomforts (previous coping mechanisms).

NURSING ASSESSMENT OF THE PATIENT WITH HEART DISEASE

The *nursing process* is the scientific method used by nurses to promote problem solving, critical thinking, care planning, analysis and data collecting. It is a flexible system which consists of four related phases: assessment, planning, implementation and evaluation. These must be completed in order to define the outcome of patient care.

Assessment is probably the most important phase of the entire process. During this phase all pertinent data about the patient (subjective and objective) are compiled through observation, history-taking, interviewing, physical examination, and examination of any pertinent laboratory findings. In order for planning, implementation and evaluation to be successfully completed, the assessment needs to be completed and organized in such a fashion that problems can be identified from it. In order for assessment to take place, a detailed health history needs to be obtained from the patient.

THE HEALTH HISTORY

There should be a specific format and procedure for obtaining and recording the subjective data the patient himself gives.

Identification of the patient

This is a brief description of the patient and includes:

1. Name
2. Sex
3. Age
4. Race and nationality
5. Marital status and next of kin
6. Address
7. Occupation
8. Source of referral
9. Chief complaint or concept of illness
10. Other pertinent characteristics

Chief complaint or concept of illness

This is the patient's description of his reason for seeking health care. It should be brief and recorded in the patient's own words. It should include the accurate description and duration of the symptoms. An appropriate way to elicit this information is to ask the question 'Why did you come to hospital?' or 'Why did you call your doctor?'

History of the present illness

The history of the present illness is a detailed description of the patient's problem. It should begin with an elaboration of the chief complaint and include a detailed history of the present problem from the time of onset to the present. The date (and time) and manner of onset and the predisposing and aggravating factors related to the onset should be elicited. The characteristics of the symptom, location, radiation, intensity, and duration should be noted. Any relieving factors and associated symptoms should be also noted. Other information of concern to the nurse is the course of the symptom(s) since onset and the effect of any treatment. Previous similar episodes will also need to be recorded.

A summary of the current state of the problem completes the history of the present illness.

Past medical history

It is important to obtain data about previous hospitalizations, illnesses, accidents, allergies and any treatment that may not be related to the present problems already identified. If it is determined that the patient is receiving specific medications, his level of knowledge and compliance should be assessed.

Review of the body systems

A systematic review of the body systems from head to toe, should elicit information about any apparent disturbance of function. Assess the patient's general state of health and his perceptive abilities. Observe for anxiety, fatigue or distress.

Skin. Texture, temperature changes, rashes, growths, photosensitivity, itching, pigmentation, dryness, sweating, characteristics of hair and nails.

Head. Headaches, migraine, convulsive seizures, vertigo, masses and any apparent trauma.

Eyes. Visual disturbances, inflammation, pain, discharge, photophobia, itching, glaucoma, cataracts, trauma, and the use of contact lenses or spectacles.

Ears. Itching, inflammation, discharge, pain, infections, hearing disturbances, and the use of hearing aids.

Nose. Inflammation, obstruction, and allergies.

Mouth and throat. Dysphagia, soreness or bleeding of gums dental problems, sore throats, and dentures.

Extremities. Numbness, parasthesia, coldness, clubbing of the fingers, and limb deformities.

Musculoskeletal system. Muscle pain, cramps, joint pain, swelling, inflammation, stiffness, fractures, back problems, arthritis, gout and the use of braces or splints.

Respiratory system. Pain, dyspnoea, shortness of breath, orthopnoea, wheezing, cough, sputum, haemoptysis, recurrent upper respiratory tract infections, bronchitis, pleurisy, pneumonia, tuberculosis, asthma, and type of tobacco and number of cigarettes smoked per day.

Cardiovascular system. Palpitations, chest pain, cyanosis, tachycardia, bradycardia, ascites, oedema, paroxysmal nocturnal dyspnoea, murmur, hypertension, phlebitis, and the presence of a permanent pacemaker.

Genito-urinary system. Dysuria, polyuria, oliguria, haematuria, pyuria, frequency, incontinence, hesitancy, sexual problems, venereal disease, vaginal discharge, and use of incontinence devices.

Gastro-intestinal tract. Appetite, weight changes, nausea, vomiting, abdominal pain, bowel habits, haemorrhoids, flatus, jaundice, and bleeding.

Life-style and activities

This should be a description of the patients daily patterns of activity. It should include information on:

Diet (e.g. normal dietary intake, calorie intake, and any supplements used).
Sleep (e.g. hours per day, sleep patterns, naps, and any sedation used).
Elimination (e.g. normal patterns, and use of any aperients).
Activities (e.g. exercise, hobbies, sports, and work).
Immunizations (e.g. childhood, polio, tetanus).
Screening procedures (e.g. medical examinations, breast examination, Pap test).

Family history

This should include the family history of diseases, ages, causes of death, and the presence of any familial diseases which are pertinent, e.g. hypertension, diabetes.

Psychosocial history

It is known that long-term significant psychological and social stress has a definite role in the development of heart disease. It is important for the nurse to obtain accurate data to help her identify problems which may affect the course of the patient's outcome. The psychosocial history should include information on the patient's education, occupation, social class, religion, social habits, interpersonal relationships, economic status, sexual habits, and methods of coping with stress.

The steps outlined above comprise the subjective part of the assessment phase. The history obtained depends very much upon the interviewing skills used by the nurse. This ability of eliciting maximal information does not always come easily to the nurse, it takes much practice and patience. The nurse needs to be relaxed and friendly in manner demonstrating a genuine concern for the patient. She should not be hurried and if she is unsure, she should ask the patient to enlarge upon his replies. The data elicited needs to be recorded accurately and carefully with the minimum of abbreviations.

The next part of the assessment phase involves the collection of objective data that are obtained from the physical examination and relevant investigations. This information frequently enlarges upon information already obtained.

Before we move on to this, it is pertinent to revise and enlarge upon some of the symptoms that are frequently encountered in the patient with cardiac problems.

SYMPTOMS AND SIGNS OF HEART DISEASE

History and general observations

As a history is being obtained from the patient, one should note particularly any symptoms that may indicate heart disease. Some general symptoms that may be associated include fever, weakness, fatigue and changes in body weight. More specific signs and symptoms of heart disease are dyspnoea, chest pain, palpitations, haemoptysis, syncope, claudication and oedema.

Dyspnoea may occur only during exertion or at rest. Orthopnoea and paroxysmal nocturnal dyspnoea may be a manifestation of left heart failure.

Chest pain needs to be carefully defined as to exact location, radiation, character, severity, duration and aggravating and relieving factors. Terms such as 'heartburn', 'wind', and 'indigestion' mean different things to different people. Therefore when analysing pain these factors should be considered.

Palpitations should be determined whether they occur on effort or at rest, and whether it begins and ends abruptly or gradually. The frequency of the attacks and the accompaniment of breathlessness or pain should be ascertained.

Haemoptysis if present, may be associated with mitral stenosis. However, the expectoration of blood is not uncommon in patients with heart disease. When there is pulmonary infection, the sputum is purulent or rusty in appearance. In pulmonary oedema, the sputum is frothy, and may be white, pink or streaked with blood.

Syncope on effort may be indicative of aortic stenosis. Syncope occurring at rest as well as during exercise may be due to heart block or other arrhythmias. However, a simple vaso-vagal faint may be caused by violent emotion or fatigue, or prolonged immobility.

Claudication may indicate peripheral arterial disease which is often accompanied by ischaemic heart disease.

Oedema. This is more correctly described as a physical sign, but the patient's observation of it may help date its onset. The milder grades of it are not noticed by the patient, but if it is more severe it may be observed in the evenings. It is usually but not invariably symmetrical in distribution, and is a manifestation of late heart failure.

Restlessness, anxiety, or inappropriate response to questioning may also indicate compromised cardiac function.

History taking
History taking improves with experience. One learns which questions to ask without 'leading' the patient. Some patients with angina may admit to chest discomfort, but deny chest pain. Some patients answer affirmatively to almost all questions concerning symptoms. The best technique is to allow the patient to relate his symptoms spontaneously. In evaluating the history, the patient's story must be believed. If the history is characteristic of organic disease it must be accepted as such, even though it may be unsupported by investigative and physical findings. Symptoms of psychogenic origin differ from those of organic disease. However, they are no less real to the patient and need to be accounted for.

Handicapped patients
Nurses should be alert to handicaps or other limitations of the patient.

They need to be familiar with the literature on the handicapped or disabled, and should try to supply the patient's particular needs, e.g. deaf people appreciate distinct rather than loud speech. They can help by providing a written list of the members of the health team. The blind need a thorough introduction to the environment with attention to the regular placement of everything they use. They also need complete verbal explanations and descriptions and the opportunity to grasp and feel as many objects as possible. Patients with serious speech impediments should be provided with pen and paper (or a 'majic-slate'). It is obvious that when the nurse cannot speak the patient's language an interpreter is needed.

It seems pertinent to mention the nurses approach to not only these patients, but to all patients as a group. It is usually the nurse who helps the patients to temporarily or permanently modify their daily activities of living. It is unfortunate that these patients are more likely to have their activities adjusted to the hospital routine, or to those of the health team upon whom these patients become dependent. The nurse should try to take into consideration previous patterns of living, and plan the patient's care accordingly.

IDENTIFYING NURSING PROBLEMS

A nursing problem is identified from the acquisition or interpretation of information and is anything of concern to either the patient or the nurse which can be helped, solved or ameliorated by nursing actions. Just by identifying a nursing problem demonstrates that there is a need for nursing care.

The nursing problem should be identified clearly and concisely. It may be medically determined, although many problems are independent of medical ones.

A nursing problem that may be identified could be:

1. Chest pain caused by a myocardial infarction. The patient is in pain, sweating and has a tachycardia.
2. Anxiety caused by hospitalization when the patient is not really aware of the reason for admission. The patient is over-talkative and restless.

When the nurse writes out a nursing problem it should include:

Identification of the problem.

Identification of the cause of the problem (if known).

Identification of how the patient is behaving in relation to the problem. (*Hunt and Marks-Moran 1980*)

When listing the problems, the nurse needs to identify priorities. This is not always feasible, as priorities may change at a later stage.

Assessment is, therefore, much more than taking a nursing history. Information has to be elicited in a number of ways, by the nurse using a variety of skills. The information that is ultimately obtained then needs to be used. It is pointless if no-one uses it constructively.

PLANNING NURSING CARE

In the assessment phase the nurse relates information about the patient to scientific knowledge regarding normal functioning and pathophysiology to arrive at a definition of the patient's problem. The tool used to move from assessment to action is called the nursing care plan. This is essential to individualized nursing care.

A nursing care plan is a detailed, written programme of action that is designed to achieve the objectives of care for a given patient. It is based on recognized nursing needs or problems and related scientific principles.

The purpose of planning care is to ensure that the best possible care is made available to the patient and to foresee and help solve future problems relating to health. The *primary nursing* method is rapidly gaining popularity. The primary nurse is responsible for a case load of patients throughout their stay in hospital. She assumes accountability for the admission history, assessment, nursing diagnosis, nursing care plans, evaluation of care, and the eventual discharge of the patient. In this way, contact between the nurse and patient is at its best, as is the continuity of care.

Nursing responsibilities

In addition to obtaining as complete assessment as possible, the nurse will have the following responsibilities:

1. Ensure that patient teaching begins at the time of admission and appears in the care plan from the start (or when unpleasant symptoms have abated).
2. Ensure that the care plans are frequently revised and updated depending on the patient's condition.

3. Ensure that the written objectives are kept clear, simple and easy to understand.
4. Consider nursing care plan conferences that include the family and patient.

IMPLEMENTING NURSING CARE

Once objectives of care are established, the nurse draws up a proposed course of action for achieving the objectives and begins the process of carrying out the plan. Implementation may include direct provision of care, counselling and teaching, and referral to other health care professionals.

Communication of instructions

If patients are to receive optimum care, instructions must be communicated successfully. Instructions should be interpreted correctly and should be written as well as verbal. The nursing care plan may be kept at a central point or at the patients bedside where they are easily accessible. It is important that other health care professionals should have access to the patients care plan. Nursing rounds and nursing care conferences help improve communication within the health care team.

Responsibility and accountability

In patient allocation one nurse is responsible and accountable for a group of patients. She decides when and how to carry out care, and she is also accountable to the nurse in charge should any care not be given to the patient.

It must also be remembered that nurses have certain legal responsibilities relating to nursing records.

EVALUATING NURSING CARE

Evaluation is the final phase of nursing care planning. It is essential for determining whether the care has been effective or not. It has three major functions:

1. Determining whether the objectives have been met.
2. Providing information for reassessment of the patient's needs.
3. Discovering which nursing actions are most consistently effective in solving a particular nursing problem.

Evaluation can be used to assess the effectiveness of the nursing care given to a particular patient, the care plans themselves, the competence of the nurse's planning and giving of care, and the overall standard of performance.

It is important that the patient's nursing problems accurately reflect the patient's needs; whether the objectives are correct (and realistic); whether the nursing actions are the most appropriate for meeting the objectives and can be carried out within the resources and time available.

TABLE 1: The nursing care plan

Problem	Objective	Care Plan	Evaluation
Chest pain due to myocardial infarction	Relief of chest pain	Give narcotic analgesic as prescribed	30 minutes – 3 hours after analgesia

THE EXTENDING ROLE OF THE NURSE

In 1974 a Joint Working Party was set up composed of officers of the DHSS and representatives of major medical and nursing professional organizations, with the following terms of reference:

'to identify areas of clinical practice in which the role of nurses (except midwives and those whose service is not the responsibility of the Departments) is extending in relation to that of doctors, taking into account the legal, ethical and training implications, with a view to establishing whether guidance to employing authorities and the profession is required'. (*DHSS 1977*)

The role of the nurse is continually developing as changes in practice and training add new functions to her normal range duties. Over and above this, however, the clinical nursing role in relation to that of the doctor may be extended in two ways: (a) by delegation by the doctor and (b) in reponse to emergencies. (*DHSS 1977*). A detailed discussion of the extended/expanded role of the nurse can be found elsewhere. (*MacGuire 1980*)

Legal implications

In an action for damages, a nurse may be held legally liable if it can be shown either that she failed to exercise the skills properly expected of her, or that she has undertaken tasks that she was not competent to perform (*DHSS 1977*). The duties and the position of the nurse should be read by each member of the profession (*RCN 1978*).

THE CLINICAL NURSE SPECIALIST/CONSULTANT

Specialization in nursing and extension of the nursing role can take place both in the assisting of patients in activities of living and in collaboration with medical advances (*McFarlane 1980*).

The Royal College of Nursing (RCN) document 'New Horizons in Clinical Nursing' (1976) shows that discussions about the development of specialized and consultant roles in nursing are still in their early stages. However, there is agreement that the clinical role of the nurse needs to be developed and that there should be career opportunities in clinical nursing comparable to those in nurse teaching and management. (*McFarlane 1980*)

REFERENCES

DHSS Health Circular HC/77/22 (1977) *Health services management: The extending role of the clinical nurse.* London: DHSS.

Henderson, V. (1960) *Basic principles of nursing care.* London: ICN.

Hunt, J.M. & Marks-Maran, D.J. (1980) *Nursing care plans.* Aylesbury: HM & M publishers.

MacGuire, J.M. (1980) *The expanded role of the nurse.* London: King's Fund.

McFarlane, J. (1980) *Essays on nursing.* London: King's Fund.

Maslow, A.H. (1970) *Motivation and personality.* New York: Harper & Row.

Roper, N., Logan, W.W. & Tierney, A.J. (1980) *The elements of nursing.* Edinburgh: Churchill Livingstone.

Roper, N., Logan, W.W. & Tierney, A.J. (1981) *Learning to use the process of nursing.* Edinburgh: Churchill Livingstone.

Royal College of Nursing (1976) *New horizons in clinical nursing.* London: RCN.

Royal College of Nursing (1978) *The duties and position of the nurse.* London: RCN.

6
Heart Failure

There is no satisfactory definition of heart failure, however, it may be defined as an abnormality of the heart beat which interferes with its activity as a pump. Failure cannot be defined simply in terms of cardiac output or *cardiac index* (output per square metre of body surface area), since this varies so widely from one individual to another and in the same individual at different times. The normal cardiac output at rest is about 5 litres per minute, yet this can be increased to about 30 litres in steady, severe exertion.

The heart maintains two circulations, systemic and pulmonary, so that two varieties of heart failure may be considered. *Left heart failure* is the most frequent and earlier type, for the commonest causes of heart disease: hypertension, aortic or mitral valve disease and ischaemic heart disease affect the left side. *Right heart failure* may occur primarily, particularly with congenital abnormalities and as a result of chronic lung disease, but it more often follows the pulmonary congestion induced by left heart failure. When there is combined left and right heart failure the condition is sometimes referred to as *congestive cardiac failure.* However, this is a term better avoided, as some understand it to mean congestion of either of these two systems, others to mean only right heart failure. When both systems are involved it should be termed combined left and right heart failure. (*Julian 1978*)

MECHANICS OF THE MYOCARDIUM

Preload (Frank–Starling mechanism)

According to this mechanism, preload is the volume of the ventricle at the end of diastole (end-diastolic volume). Starling's law states that the force with which the heart contracts depends on the extent to which it has been stretched prior to contraction. Therefore, an increase in end-diastolic volume (preload) is followed by a more powerful contraction that improves ventricular emptying. In the normal heart, the Frank–Starling mechanism operates mainly to match the stroke outputs of the two ventricles. However, in heart failure, this mechanism plays an important part in sustaining the cardiac output. Vasodilator drugs can help reduce the atrial pressures with no fall in the stroke volume.

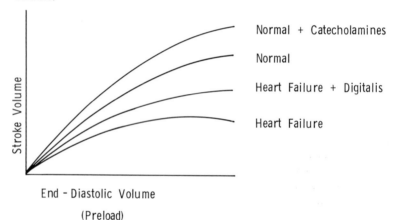

Fig. 54. *The relationship between stroke volume and end-diastolic volume.*

Afterload

Afterload refers to the force that the ventricle must develop during systole in order to eject the stroke volume. A fall in preload may reduce afterload. In the failing heart, vasodilators produce a fall in resistance (or impedance), which reduces the work demanded of the left ventricle.

Myocardial contractility (Inotropic state)

Changes in myocardial contractility can alter the performance of the ventricle. Under normal circumstances, myocardial contractility is largely dependent upon the activity of the cardiac sympathetic nerves, but it can be augmented by circulating catecholamines, tachycardia, cardiac glycosides, isoprenaline, and calcium. Myocardial contractility is depressed by hypoxia, acidosis, quinidine, procainamide, and many other drugs. When a portion of ventricular myocardium becomes necrosed the total ventricular performance is depressed. (*Braunwald et al 1976*)

Causes. Most types of heart disease result in a mechanical stress upon the heart. The two most common general types of mechanical cardiac stress are that resulting from an increased resistance to ventricular emptying or increased afterload (pressure overload) and that resulting from increased ventricular filling or increased preload (volume overload).

In the majority of patients with a chronic pressure load or a chronic volume load on the left ventricle, heart failure is preceded by myocardial dysfunction and then failure.

Pressure overload. Increased afterload (pressure overload) of the left ventricle is seen in patients with hypertension or aortic stenosis. The basic reaction of the myocardium is to contract more forcefully, but more slowly. The myocardium also hypertrophies (concentric hypertrophy), in which there is marked thickening of the left ventricular wall, including the septum, but there is no increase in the size of the left ventricular cavity.

Volume overload. In left ventricular preload (volume overload), the ventricle hypertrophies (eccentric hypertrophy), in which the ventricular chamber and the left ventricular wall increase in size proportionally.

LEFT HEART FAILURE

The left heart may fail gradually or acutely.

Aetiology
The common causes of left heart failure are:

Hypertension
Aortic stenosis and incompetence
Mitral incompetence

Myocardial infarction

Hypertrophic obstructive cardiomyopathy (HOCM)

Clinical features

When the left ventricle fails it is unable to fully expel its contents, thus the diastolic pressure in the left ventricle increases, followed by an increase of pressure in the left atrium and pulmonary veins. When the rise in pressure becomes sufficiently high, fluid is forced out of the circulation into the alveoli, and *oedema* of the lungs occur. These mechanical effects of failure of the left ventricle are termed as *pulmonary venous congestion*. Finally, *bronchospasm* is often a marked feature, and when prominent, the condition is called *cardiac asthma*.

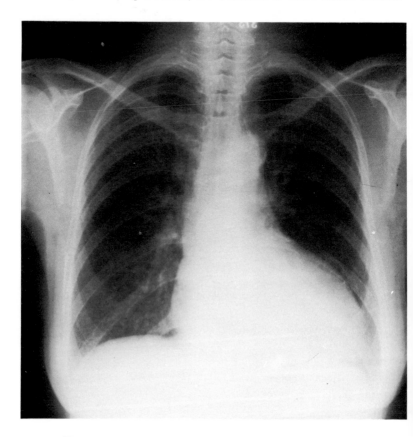

Fig. 55. *X-ray of the heart with left ventricular hypertrophy.*

Other features include:

Dyspnoea (breathlessness) on exertion.
Orthopnoea (breathlessness on lying flat).
Tachypnoea (increased frequency of respirations).
Paroxysmal nocturnal dyspnoea.
Acute pulmonary oedema is also present.

Pulmonary congestion may lead to the physical signs of cyanosis, and sometimes hydrothorax.

Pulses. Alternate large and small pulses (pulsus alternans), are characteristic.

Auscultation. *Basal crepitations* are commonly heard in pulmonary congestion. A *third heart sound* is heard which is caused by rapid ventricular filling.

Investigations
Blood pressure. A fall in blood pressure in a patient with hypertension is often an early indicator of failure.

Chest X-ray. This may show pulmonary venous congestion, and sometimes pulmonary oedema.

ECG. This may be of value; although it does not provide direct evidence of left heart failure, it may give evidence of increasing left ventricular hypertrophy or ischaemia.

RIGHT HEART FAILURE

The right heart fails more readily, and is commonly secondary to left heart failure. In fact, pure right heart failure is uncommon.

Aetiology
The common causes of right heart failure are:

Chronic lung disease.
Tricuspid valve disease.
Pulmonary valve disease.

Clinical features
When the right ventricle fails, the pressure rises in the right atrium,

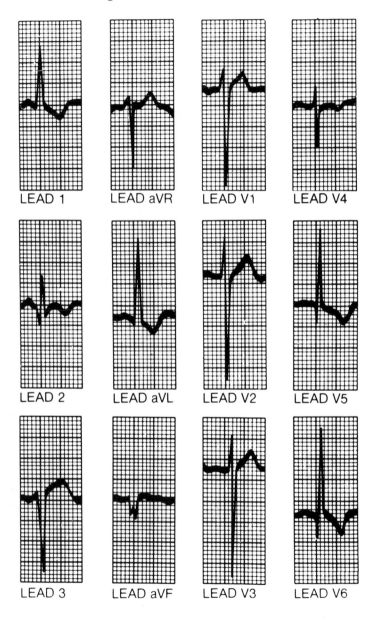

Fig. 56. *Electrocardiogram of left ventricular hypertrophy.*

the venae cavae, the hepatic and the systemic veins. The effects of systemic venous congestion: engorged veins, enlarged and tender liver, and oedema can be easily observed. An increased venous pressure occurs in the *jugular pulse* known as the *jugular venous pressure* (JVP). Other features include:

Dyspnoea, at first on exertion, later at rest.

Cyanosis is common, partly due to poor oxygenation of the blood passing through the oedematous lung and partly due to peripheral stagnation.

Nausea and vomiting due to gastric congestion, and anorexia and fatigue occur.

Weakness, insomnia, loss of memory, mental confusion and *oliguria* are all due to the diminished blood supply to the vital organs.

Pleural effusion and *ascites* are additional features of massive cardiac oedema.

Signs of the disease causing either the right or left heart failure which so often precedes it, may also be present.

Precipitating factors in heart failure

Heart failure may be precipitated or exacerbated by:

Anaemia
Atrial fibrillation
Myocardial infarction
Pregnancy
Pulmonary embolism
Excessive sodium intake

TREATMENT

It is important to treat the cause of heart failure first. Treatment of heart failure itself must be started as soon as it is recognized. The three most important measures are rest, digitalis and diuretic therapy.

Rest

Reduced physical activity is an important way to make the best use of a limited cardiac output. The patient should understand that physical and mental rest has positive advantages. It does not necessarily imply complete bed rest and, unless the failure is acute or severe, the patient should be allowed to care for himself. Movement of the legs, and short periods out of bed should be encouraged to limit the dangers of venous thrombosis and pulmonary embolism. Sedation throughout the day and a hypnotic at night often ensure adequate rest and alleviate mood changes which often accompany enforced rest. An excellent alternative to bed rest is a comfortable, high-backed armchair; many patients find this supportive and so rest and sleep more easily. Early mobilization should be aimed for once the patient's physical state permits.

Digitalis

This is indicated in many cases of heart failure. Digitalis is one of a group of drugs collectively known as the cardiac glycosides. It is the single most important drug in the treatment of heart failure. In therapeutic doses it has no effect on the normal heart, but in failure it improves the contractility of the myocardium (positive inotropic effect), increases the cardiac output (which produces diuresis), and lowers venous pressure. The principles of digitalis therapy are discussed on p. 257.

Diuretics

Digitalis produces its diuretic effect by increasing effective blood flow through the kidney. If this is insufficient in treating oedema, then diuretics (drugs which have a direct effect on the kidney) are indicated. High potency diuretics such as frusemide and ethacrynic acid have a rapid action and are useful in an emergency. However, in moderate heart failure and for long-term maintenance, thiazide diuretics are usually added. Diuretic therapy greatly improves the progress of heart failure, but it must be carefully monitored. The principles of diuretic therapy are discussed on p. 259.

Vasodilators

Vasodilator drugs are becoming of greater importance in the treatment of heart failure. These drugs improve cardiac output and decrease venous pressure. There are several available vasodilators which vary in their site of action. The commonest ones in use are hydralazine and prazosin. Vasodilators are discussed in greater detail on p. 265.

ACUTE LEFT VENTRICULAR FAILURE (LVF)

Acute LVF (paroxysmal dyspnoea and acute pulmonary oedema) is an emergency. The clinical features include breathlessness at rest, cyanosis, and a dry cough. At a later stage the patient often coughs up blood-stained froth. Urgent treatment is required.

The patient is more comfortable sitting up. Diamorphine should be given as this relieves the dyspnoea by relieving anxiety, peripheral venous dilatation, and reducing sensitivity of the respiratory centre to reflex stimulation from the stiff congested lungs. Aminophylline administered slowly intravenously, will lower the venous pressure and relieve the bronchospasm. The hypoxia of acute LVF is larely due to ventilation-perfusion imbalance, therefore oxygen is beneficial. Intravenous frusemide is also of value in relieving pulmonary oedema. Digoxin is also given intravenously, provided there are no contra-indications. Venesection of 500 ml of blood may reduce venous return. However, this may be difficult to carry out.

Nitroprusside is a potent vasodilator which is useful in selected patients. It is given intravenously, and has a rapid onset of action. It is particularly useful in those patients with myocardial infarction and left ventricular failure. (*Opie 1980*)

NURSING CARE

The main aims of nursing care are to reduce the workload of the heart, provide a stress-free environment, and observe the efficiency of the drug therapy being used. Nursing care plans should be devised with these objectives in mind.

The nurse should allay anxiety in these patients by explaining what the problem is and how the patient and nurse can work together with the aim of a complete recovery.

Obese patients will require a reducing diet, and all patients in failure should be encouraged to eat small, easily digestible, evenly spaced out meals. They should be advised to rest afterwards. A low sodium diet has now been generally superseded by diuretic therapy. However, some restriction of sodium intake is desirable, and the nurse can advise them to avoid salt at meals and to avoid obviously salty foods. There is no reason to restrict fluid intake when sodium retention is eliminated by diet and diuretics. (*Karliner 1981*)

Smoking should be avoided. A mild aperient or suppository may be given to avoid constipation. The patient will most likely find it easier to use a bedside commode rather than a bedpan. Because of diuretic therapy, male patients may find it easier to stand out of bed and use a urinal.

Patients in acute LVF are usually very anxious or frightened and need a lot of psychological support. Diamorphine and frequent sedation often relieves this anxiety. Oxygen therapy also appears to be beneficial, and the highest available concentration may be used if there are no contraindications. These patients are often most comfortable sitting up, either in bed or in a chair.

REFERENCES

Braunwald, E., Ross, J. & Sonnenblick, E.H. (1976) *Mechanisms of contraction in the normal and failing heart.* Boston: Little Brown & Co.

Julian, D.G. (1978) *Cardiology.* London: Baillière Tindall.

Karliner, J.S. (1981) *Congestive heart failure: pathophysiology and treatment.* In *Coronary Care* (Ed: J.S. Karliner & G. Gregoratos), New York: Churchill Livingstone.

Opie, L.H. (1980) *Drugs and the heart.* London: *Lancet* (publication).

7
Ischaemic
Heart Disease

INTRODUCTION

Ischaemic heart disease (IHD) is the major cause of death in the Western world. There are some 150 000 deaths from IHD in the United Kingdom (UK) each year: 55 000 of these occur in people aged less than seventy years, and approximately 100 000 of these take place outside hospital. The majority are sudden in that they happen within one hour of the onset of symptoms. Nine out of every ten deaths from IHD are a result of ventricular fibrillation (VF). (*Adgey 1980*)

DEFINITION

The term *ischaemic heart disease* is used to describe cardiac disease due to obstruction of the coronary arteries by atheroma. It is synonymous with the terms *coronary heart disease* and *atherosclerotic heart disease*. The term *coronary artery disease* is *not* synonymous with ischaemic heart disease.

Coronary thrombosis is used to describe the occlusion of a coronary artery by thrombus.
Coronary occlusion is used to describe the occlusion of the coronary artery by any cause.
Myocardial infarction is used to indicate necrosis of a portion of heart muscle (myocardium) as a result of inadequate blood supply.

INCIDENCE

The incidence of IHD increases with age. It has its maximum incidence in males between the ages of 45 and 55 years, and in females between 55 and 65 years of age. Under the age of 45, IHD is more than ten times as common in males as in females; between 45 and 60 it is twice as common in males; in the older age groups the incidence is approximately equal in both sexes. But the disease is becoming more common affecting both sexes at progressively earlier ages.

THE CORONARY CIRCULATION: NORMAL FUNCTION

The anatomy of the coronary arteries has already been described.

The coronary arteries are compressed by the contracting myocardium during systole so that the resistance to flow at that time is sharply increased. Consequently, coronary blood flow occurs mainly during diastole. Because the force of contraction of the right ventricle is much less than of the left, flow in the right coronary artery is less disturbed by systole during which there is relatively more coronary blood flow to the right ventricle than to the left. Coronary blood flow is largely determined by the calibre of the coronary arteries themselves. According to Poiseuille's equation, flow is dependent directly on pressure differences but related to the fourth power of the radius. Because aortic diastolic pressure is also a determinant of coronary blood flow, a doubling of this would result in a doubling of the coronary flow, whereas a doubling of the radius of the coronary arteries leads to a sixteen-fold increase in coronary flow. Lack of oxygen due to hypoxia or anaemia causes a profound increase in flow (up to five-fold), being the most potent coronary vasodilator. An excess of carbon dioxide and lactic acid causes only slight vasodilation (unlike the cerebral vessels where CO_2 is an important vasodilator). Changes in tissue oxygen tension are probably responsible for most of the variations in coronary blood flow.

Normally, the heart extracts a high and relatively fixed percentage of the oxygen from coronary arterial blood. Since increased oxygen extraction is thus not possible, augmented myocardial oxygen demands must be met by increases in coronary blood flow. This is largely dependent upon the ability of the coronary arteries to increase their diameter.

ATHEROMA

The term atheroma describes a disorder of arteries which begins with patchy fatty deposits in the arterial wall, and later leads to a fibrous reaction and the formation of plaques. As these plaques enlarge, extend and multiply they can cause stenosis and eventually occlusion of the affected vessel, or they may weaken the vessel wall and cause dilatation complicated by thrombosis or rupture. Alternatively, a plaque may ulcerate and discharge its contents into the arterial lumen to give lipid emboli, leaving a rough surface which provides a base for thrombus to form.

There are several conflicting theories about the pathogenesis of atheroma. The most widely held theory is that, due to metabolic abnormalities, the chemical constitution of the blood is in some way altered so as to lead to the deposition of fatty substances in the arterial wall.

By the time atheromatous disease becomes apparent it is locally very severe and usually widespread.

Experimental studies in animals have shown that atheroma can be induced by cholesterol feeding. However, the lesions produced differ from those in the humans. *(McMichael 1979)*

Atheroma cannot be diagnosed on clinical grounds until IHD produces manifest symptoms and signs. However, an increased liability to atherosclerosis can be suspected in individuals exhibiting the signs of hypercholesterolaemia such as xanthomatous deposits.

AETIOLOGICAL FACTORS

Atheroma of the coronary circulation is almost always the underlying pathological process of ischaemic heart disease. Most evidence on risk factors in atheroma is based on research into heart disease. The factors that identify individuals at increased risk from heart disease (IHD) were suspected decades ago. Studies have consistently shown three factors to be powerful predictors of IHD. These are:

1. Plasma cholesterol level
2. Blood pressure level
3. Cigarette consumption

According to the Framingham Study, the risk of IHD is one-third of the 'standard risk' in the subjects with a low plasma cholesterol level, normal blood pressure and who are non-smokers. It is ten times the 'standard risk' in subjects with an elevated plasma cholesterol level, increased blood pressure and who smoke cigarettes. *(Kannel et al 1964)*

Other specific risk factors

Major. High saturated fat diet; Glucose intolerance (Diabetes mellitus); Obesity.

Minor. Oral contraceptives; Sedentary living; Personality type; Psychosocial.

Risk factors such as age, sex and familial history are non-modifiable, while others are modifiable.

Although by definition each risk factor associates positively with the risk of IHD, it by no means follows that risk factors are causal. It must be stressed that *association does not necessarily imply causation.* For example, the evidence available so far does not allow us to conclude that smoking causes IHD. The association between cigarette smoking and IHD is weak relative to that for lung cancer and several other malignancies. On the other hand, it cannot be conclusively ruled out that physical exertion might *hasten* death from IHD. (*Burch 1980*)

LIPIDS

The plasma lipids, composed mainly of cholesterol, triglyceride, phospholipid, and free fatty acids, are substances that are insoluble in water and therefore require a carrier to circulate from one tissue to another. These carriers are the lipoproteins which, as the term implies, are compounds of protein and lipid.

The important lipids in IHD are plasma cholesterol and triglycerides. There is a high incidence of IHD in individuals with elevated plasma lipid levels, particularly if they have familial hyperlipoproteinaemia.

There are four major classes of lipoprotein:

Chylomicron
VLDL (very low density lipoprotein)
LDL (low density lipoprotein)
HDL (high density lipoprotein)

Each contain varying proportions of cholesterol, triglycerides, phospholipid and protein. HDL has the least portion of cholesterol and triglycerides, while VLDL has the greatest portion of these.

There has been interest in the HDL or αcholesterol fraction. This has been found to correlate inversely with the risk of IHD, and must therefore behave differently from the rest of the circulating cholesterol.

HYPERLIPIDAEMIA

Increases in the concentration of one or more of the lipoproteins constitutes a particular type of hyperlipidaemia (hyperlipoprotein-aemia).

There are various systems of classification but the most widely used is the Fredrickson classification, which is based on electrophoresis.

Types IIa and IIb and Type III are closely associated with coronary atherosclerosis. Type IV also seems probable as being relevant to coronary disease.

THE DIETARY FAT THEORY

Much controversy exists about dietary fats and IHD. It is thought that a reduction of the level of plasma cholesterol by diet, drugs or other means will lead to a reduced incidence of IHD. This so-called *lipid hypothesis* (high-fat diet → high plasma cholesterol → atheroma → IHD) is based on the assumption that raised concentrations of plasma cholesterol increase the severity of the atheromatous lesions, and may even be a factor in their development. However, this remains very uncertain. (*McMichael 1979; Thompson 1980a*)

It would appear that cholesterol-reducing measures have not been proven. Yet many committees have recommended a reduction in dietary saturated fat (dairy produce, meat and meat products) and also an increase in polyunsaturated fat (seeds, grains, nuts and the oils extracted from them, and from greens and other vegetables). (Joint Working Party of the Royal College of Physicians of London and the British Cardiac Society 1976; US Senate Committee on Nutrition 1977.) Others would argue that a high intake of sucrose is more likely a causative factor than saturated fats, and this may well be true. (*Yudkin 1972*)

Obesity

It is only fairly gross levels of obesity that appear to matter. Weight loss appears to be beneficial as it is often associated with a change in blood pressure.

Glucose intolerance

Diabetics are at very high risk from atheromatous disease but the risk in the general population appears to be confined to the very top of the distribution of glucose intolerance.

Family history

IHD often occurs in several members of the same family and there can be little doubt that hereditary factors are involved. This could be genetic and/or it could be that behaviour associated with coronary risk is learnt within the family.

Physical activity

Studies seem to show that leisure exercise does have a protective effect.

Personality

The so called type A personality (aggressive, competitive men with a great sense of time urgency, who set themselves multiple deadlines and speak in a characteristic staccato manner) are at increased risk.

Nearly all these risk factors are subject to great controversy. It may be that the type A personality will receive much more attention in the near future. Whereas obesity, diet and even cigarette smoking are being challenged as risk factors, it is probable that high blood pressure will emerge as the most important risk factor.

POSSIBLE FACTORS INFLUENCING THE DEVELOPMENT OF IHD OR ITS COMPLICATIONS

These include:

Decreased physical activity and fitness
Type A personality
Psychosocial tension
Sucrose intake
Water softness
Occupation (e.g. doctors)
Social overcrowding
Income, living standards
Tachycardia at rest
Abnormal ECG at rest or during exercise
Sticky platelets
Elevated haematocrit

New ideas regarding the recognition and treatment of certain aspects of IHD are continually emerging. Unfortunately, less progress has been made in the prevention of IHD. Current methods of prevention have not gained universal popular acceptance and the value of this approach is therefore limited.

EFFECTS OF ISCHAEMIA

Inadequate myocardial oxygenation induced by the atherosclerotic process results in abnormalities of the biochemical, electrical, and mechanical functioning of the heart.

Intracellular lactate is formed, accumulates and is eventually released into coronary sinus blood. This is, to some degree, detected by cardiac enzyme estimation.

Ischaemia alters the electrical properties of the heart, the most characteristic early changes in the ECG being those of the repolarization process (inversion of T waves and displacement of ST segments). Electrical instability leading to ventricular tachycardia (VT) and fibrillation (VF) is another consequence of myocardial ischaemia.

The contractile function of the myocardium is markedly impaired. Necrosis causes an irreversible loss of function with eventual scar formation.

CLINICAL PRESENTATION OF IHD

Ischaemic heart disease includes the clinical syndromes of:

Angina
Acute myocardial infarction
Sudden death

Each of these syndromes is almost invariably associated with the presence of advanced atherosclerosis. This usually involves at least one and often two or three main coronary arteries. However, not everyone who has severe and extensive atherosclerosis will develop clinical IHD.

ANGINA

Angina pectoris occurs when the oxygen demand of the myocardium exceeds its supply. Pain characteristic of angina is usually easily recognized by four characteristic features: site, character, relation to increased heart work and duration.

The site of the pain

The pain is felt in the retrosternal region. It radiates upwards to the throat and lower jaw and is accompanied by heaviness or numbness of the left arm, right arm, or both arms, and sometimes tingling of the fingers. It may also radiate to the back or epigastrium. Patients have been described with anginal pain occurring only in the left wrist, or between the scapulae.

The character of the pain
The pain is described as 'choking', 'tight', 'squeezing', 'constricting', 'burning' or 'like a weight'. The pain is rarely stabbing. Although it is not usually severe it causes much anxiety and distress, the patient often saying that he 'cannot get his breath'. Many patients suffering from angina attribute their pain and discomfort to 'indigestion'.

The relationship of pain to increased heart work
Typically the pain of angina is precipitated by exercise or emotion. If exercise is responsible, it is nearly always that of walking, particularly up hill, more easily so after a heavy meal or in cold weather. Emotion is an important provoking factor; angina often develops during sexual intercourse and may be induced by anger and irritation. It is pertinent to note that many patients experience angina which is induced by watching television.

The duration of the pain
If the patient is exercising, the pain makes him stop; it is relieved within five minutes of rest or removal of the causative stimulus. If glyceryl trinitrate (nitroglycerin) is used properly, it can relieve the pain faster than rest alone. The duration is rarely less than 30 seconds or more than 15 minutes.

Anginal attacks at rest
Recent studies with continuous ECG and haemodynamic monitoring have shown that anginal attacks at rest characterized by ST segment elevation or depression were never preceded by haemodynamic changes. Indeed, the pattern observed was very similar to that seen during experimental, transient coronary occlusion. (*Maseri 1981*)

Other accompaniments of angina
Some patients complain of dyspnoea accompanying the anginal pain. Other patients with angina feel faint or dizzy and syncope occurs occasionally. Some patients, presumably because the pain is very severe, also sweat and have nausea, very occasionally with vomiting.

TYPES OF ANGINA

Stable angina

This occurs over a long period of time in the same pattern of onset, duration, and intensity of symptoms.

Unstable angina

The frequency, intensity, and duration of symptoms increase as the atherosclerotic process progresses. Many patients with this type of angina will infarct within 3 to 18 months after the onset. Other names attributed to this syndrome include: acute coronary insufficiency, prodromal syndrome, and preinfarction syndrome.

Prinzmetal angina

This is chest pain at rest due to coronary artery spasm which causes transient ST segment *elevation* during pain. The ECG changes disappear once the pain subsides. Arrhythmias are often associated with this type of angina. It is also known as variant angina.

Angina decubitus

This is chest pain that occurs in the recumbent position, relieved by sitting or standing. It usually implies the involvement of the three coronary arteries.

Nocturnal angina

This occurs only at night, and not necessarily in the recumbent position. It may be possibly provoked by vivid dreams.

Intractable angina

This is chronic chest pain that is physically incapacitating, and refractory to medical treatment.

INVESTIGATIONS

ECG

It is important to realize that the resting ECG is normal in many patients with symptomatic IHD. Changes in the resting ECG result from myocardial effects occurring relatively late in the disease. There may be non-specific changes such as flattening or inversion of T waves in the leads in which they are normally upright. Also, there may be the changes of previous infarction with Q waves. Finally, there may be signs of a conduction defect: varying degrees of atrioventricular block, or isolated right or left bundle branch block. If the patient is seen during an attack, an ECG will show (usually) well-marked abnormalities: horizontal or downward sloping ST segment depression. These changes may be provoked by an exercise test.

Exercise (stress) testing

Electrocardiographic ST segment displacement is a characteristic response to ischaemia and occurs during and immediately following an exercise test. The patient exercises on steps, a bicycle ergometer or a treadmill. A 12 lead ECG is obtained during exercise and on three occasions during the first 10 minutes of rest. A positive exercise test is generally defined as a horizontal depression of the ST segment of 0.5 mm or more below the base-line, or a downward sloping ST segment. The depression is of the *square wave* or *plateau* type. ST segment depression which slopes upwards is referred to as a junctional change. The latter slopes upwards from the J point and should not be regarded as evidence of ischaemia as they are often seen in normal individuals with tachycardia.

The exercise test remains the best available method for screening a population to determine the presence of coronary disease, and with the current emphasis on prevention of IHD it is being widely used.

Pacing

Stress by cardiac pacing has the advantage that the patient is usually not aware of the stimulus so that false positive results are less of a problem.

Nuclear imaging

An isotope (e.g. thallium–201) is introduced intravenously and a gamma camera used to follow its passage through the myocardium. A scan is usually done first on exercise and then again later when the thallium is redistributed within the myocardium. If a perfusion defect is present only on exercise then that area of myocardium only becomes ischaemic on exercise.

Coronary arteriography

This is of great value in establishing the presence or absence of atheroma, and estimating the severity of the obstructive lesion which may be present. The investigation is essential in patients being considered for coronary artery surgery. Left ventriculography is also undertaken to assess myocardial function.

In the majority of patients, a confident diagnosis of angina is made from the medical history. Physical examination and investigations other than those noted are of comparatively little value. It is important to exclude predisposing factors such as hypothyroidism, chronic nephritis, diabetes and hypertension.

Angina may need to be differentiated from left infra-mammary pain, 'indigestion', hiatus hernia and cervical spondylosis. Stabbing pains occurring on effort, below the nipple and persistent aches in the same region, unrelated to effort, are common and are most unlikely to be due to IHD. They are very common in those with anxiety neurosis.

TREATMENT

Angina is one of the commonest features of IHD. Chronic angina with predictable precipitating factors (stable angina) is usually quite well managed. The patient should be kept pain-free by optimal use of drugs. However, if angina remains a serious problem, coronary artery surgery should be considered.

Treatment generally consists of risk factor control, symptomatic relief, and prophylaxis. Coronary artery surgery will probably need to be considered at a later date.

Risk factor control

Hypertension. Persistent hypertension increases the demand for oxygen by the heart, apart from the added risks to the coronary arteries (increasing atheroma). Hypertension, therefore, needs to be controlled, because of the possible beneficial effect on the angina.

Cigarette smoking. Cigarette smokers should be advised to stop or at least reduce their consumption.

Hyperlipidaemia. It has not been shown that the control of hyperlipidaemia by diet and drugs has any beneficial effect on either the symptoms or the prognosis. There is no proof that clofibrate (Atromid–S) improves patients' symptoms.

Obesity. It would seem beneficial to advise obese patients to lose weight.

Underlying heart disease may produce angina, e.g. aortic stenosis, anaemia, cardiomyopathy and thyrotoxicosis.

GENERAL MEASURES

The patient may have to modify his lifestyle. Physical exercise to a point short of precipitating pain should be encouraged, but those activities which regularly provoke pain, despite adequate drug therapy, should be avoided. The patient may have to walk more slowly and avoid heavy meals. He may have to wear warm clothes as cold weather may precipitate angina.

Patients (e.g. manual labourers) may need to change their occupation. Drivers who hold HGV and PSV licenses and airline pilots are obliged to inform the licensing authorities and must change jobs.

The patient should be advised to avoid sudden strenuous effort, and to carefully plan his daily programme in advance in order to minimize anxiety and stress. Anxiety provoking situations need to be avoided and this advice needs to be stressed to the family, and spouse in particular.

SYMPTOMATIC RELIEF

During the acute attack of angina, the patient should be advised to stand still or sit down as soon as discomfort starts. Relief may be hastened if oral glyceryl trinitrate is taken.

Glyceryl trinitrate

This is a short-acting nitrate which has been used for a great many years and is still the most valuable drug in the treatment of angina. Its main action seems to be on peripheral vessels causing lowered peripheral resistance, venous return and blood pressure; thus heart work is reduced.

Glyceryl trinitrate (nitroglycerin or trinitrin) should be taken sublingually as it is ineffective when swallowed. It has a rapid onset of action, and its effect persists for up to 45 minutes. The important point about glyceryl trinitrate is that it should be used to *prevent* angina. This advice is not given often enough to patients, who are often frightened that the drug may be addictive or harmful. Patients need to be advised that the drug is *good* for them, not bad. It must be impressed upon them that the pain is *bad* for them. The drug is effective in preventing attacks and stops them usually within a minute.

It is important that information about glyceryl trinitrate is given to the patient. Because the drug is volatile and vapourises, it needs to be stored in vapour-proof bottles. For this reason, there should be *no* cotton wool in the bottles. If the patient keeps the drug on him at all times, the tablets need to be kept in an outside pocket (i.e. jacket pocket) and not in a shirt pocket, etc. The patient should be encouraged to always keep a supply of the drug near at hand. Tablets should be discarded after two months as they are not as effective.

The patient should be instructed to take a tablet when he feels the pain coming on. When first starting on the tablets it is advisable that the patient is sitting or reclining as syncope occasionally occurs from a sudden fall in blood pressure. The tablet can be sucked or chewed. For a rapid effect the patient can crunch the tablet between his teeth. Once relief has been obtained the remainder of the tablet can be discarded or swallowed.

The patient should be warned about headaches which often accompany the use of this drug. It should be explained that this is harmless and often subsides with continued use. The patient should be advised to discard the tablet if he feels a headache coming on.

Patients need to be reassured that they can take as many tablets as they need throughout the day, without any harm.

PROPHYLAXIS

Beta-adrenergic blocking agents
These drugs have revolutionized the medical management of angina. Their chief beneficial effect is to reduce the oxygen requirement of the heart by reducing heart rate and velocity of contraction.

Propanolol (Inderal) is the most widely used drug. It should be taken about four times a day for optimum effect in angina. Sustained release and long-acting preparations, such as propranolol (Inderal-LA) and atenolol (Tenormin), can be taken once-daily.

Long-acting nitrates
Certain nitrate compounds, particularly isosorbide dinitrate (Isordil, Cedocard), are very effective. Long-acting and sustained release preparations (Cedocard Retard) and intravenous preparations are particularly useful for coronary artery spasm.

Glyceryl trinitrate (GTN) ointment, or paste, has recently been made available. The beneficial effects are much longer-lasting than the sublingual form.

Other drugs
Nifedipine (Adalat) is an antianginal agent which probably has its major effect through vasodilatation. It is a potent and long-acting drug. For the relief of pain, the capsule may be bitten and the contents held in

the mouth. Unwanted effects are similar to those of the nitrates (headache and dizziness), but it is generally well tolerated.

Perhexilene (Pexid) and verapamil (Cordilox) have been used, and although effective, have not gained widespread acceptance. Dipyridamole (Persantin) is no longer recommended in the management of angina.

Prostacyclin has recently been shown to prevent platelet aggregation. Coronary and systemic vasodilator effects also indicate an acute beneficial effect of prostacyclin on angina pectoris. (*Bergman et al 1981*)

CORONARY ARTERY SURGERY

In a large proportion of patients, angina can be relieved by coronary bypass surgery. This is done by bypassing the obstructions with homologous saphenous vein grafts from the aorta to the distal coronary arteries. Patients which should be considered for surgery include those with symptoms that are not easily controlled by medical therapy. Survival is prolonged in severe proximal three-vessel disease and left main-stem disease at least.

It is generally accepted that symptoms are relieved and the quality of life improved by surgery in approximately 90% of patients. Despite good surgical results and a dramatic improvement in the quality of life, the risks (although low) must be weighed against potential benefits. (*Cattell and Balcon 1981*)

PROGNOSIS

The prognosis of angina is not poor; mortality in patients with angina is about 5% per year. Most patients with angina live a normal or near normal life, and every effort should be made to encourage this. It should be realised that the patients' symptoms will vary from time to time, becoming worse in winter and improving the subsequent summer.

ACUTE MYOCARDIAL INFARCTION

The most important clinical manifestations of IHD are acute myocardial infarction and sudden death. Identified heart attacks occur in about 0.5 – 1.0% of the population each year. Between a third and a half of all cardiac deaths occur in medically unattended situations, the rest under observation in hospital.

The diagnosis of acute myocardial infarction is based on the history aided by the electrocardiogram. Cardiac enzyme tests are used to confirm the diagnosis or, quantitatively, to indicate the extent of myocardial damage.

PATHOLOGY

The essential pathological feature is myocardial necrosis. This may result from occlusion of a coronary artery but sometimes occurs in its absence. The infarcted area is at first red owing to extravasation of the red cells (infarct means 'stuffed in' with red cells). The area later appears pale as the necrotic muscle swells and squeezes out the extravasated blood. Finally, the infarcted area is replaced by fibrous scar tissue.

An infarction may be *subendocardial*, in which case the necrotic tissue is on the endocardial surface; *intramural*, or confined to the interior of the myocardium; *epicardial*, or involving just the epicardial surface; or *transmural*, involving the full thickness of the ventricular wall, the endocardium, and the epicardium.

Infarction may be located in the *anterior* region if the left anterior descending artery is occluded (where it may involve the septum and papillary muscles); in the *posterior* region of the left ventricle if the left circumflex artery is occluded; and in the *inferior* (diaphragmatic) region if the right coronary artery is occluded. Because of the frequency of involvement of the left ventricle, classification according to location is usually in reference to this chamber. Each classification is further broken down to designate the particular section of the wall involved: *lateral* or *septal*. A septal infarction involves the interventricular area of the anterior, posterior, or inferior wall, and a lateral infarct involves the far side of the wall of the chamber.

The factors leading to occlusion of the diseased vessel by thrombosis are not fully understood, although it is known that the 'stickiness' of platelets is increased in patients with IHD.

HAEMODYNAMICS

Left ventricular dysfunction occurs in most patients after myocardial infarction although it is not always clinically apparent. In left ventricular failure (LVF) with increased end-diastolic pressures the clinical picture of pulmonary congestion develops.

The poor perfusion caused by reduced cardiac output may be followed by shock, with hypotension, oliguria and acidosis. Oliguria results from reduced renal perfusion following low cardiac output and hypotension. This condition is sometimes called 'cardiogenic shock', and it is usually fatal.

CLINICAL FEATURES

Chest pain

This is the dominant symptom in acute myocardial infarction. The typical prolonged retrosternal pain is described as 'crushing', 'vice-like', 'tight' or 'constricting'. In general terms, the pain is usually greater than half an hour in duration. Sometimes the 'pain' is described as discomfort. Often there is a history of angina which has increased in severity and frequency prior to the attack. However, unlike the pain of angina, it is seldom associated with exertion and it is unrelieved by rest or glyceryl trinitrate, often persisting for several hours. In addition to retrosternal pain, referred pain may radiate into either or both arms, or towards the neck or lower jaw. Acute myocardial infarction without pain has been claimed to occur more often in elderly people.

The chest pain of acute myocardial infarction is frequently accompanied by nausea, vomiting, faintness, sweating, palpitations or a syncopal episode. Marked anxiety is a common feature.

Once the pain is controlled the general appearance improves and often, within a few hours, the patient looks relatively well.

Pulses

The arterial pulse may be normal in volume and rate, although sinus tachycardia is common as a result of pain, anxiety or heart failure. Sinus bradycardia may be present, especially when the infarction affects the inferior wall: increased vagal tone is usually responsible. However, bradycardia may be a result of heart block.

Blood pressure

Initially, the blood pressure is usually normal, although a slight rise often occurs. The level usually falls progressively over a period of 24 hours. Occasionally, there may be a sharp fall of blood pressure at the onset of the infarction. If this becomes severe and associated with a low cardiac output, cardiogenic shock occurs, which is usually fatal.

Auscultation

The heart sounds are often soft. A third sound suggests heart failure. Occasionally a loud systolic murmur appears, due to a rupture of the ventricular septum or of a papillary muscle. A faint pericardial rub is sometimes heard. A loud rub appears after the third day and this indicates generalized pericarditis.

Basal crepitations due to pulmonary oedema are common but usually of little importance.

Temperature

During the first few days there is usually a fever, seldom exceeding 38 °C. The pyrexia is often accompanied by a leucocytosis and raised erythrocyte sedimentation rate (ESR), representing a reaction to myocardial necrosis.

ECG

Three pathophysiological events occur, either in sequence or simultaneously, in an acute myocardial infarction: ischaemia, injury, and infarction. The electrocardiographic manifestations of these processes involve changes in the T wave (ischaemia), ST segments (injury), and Q waves (infarction).

A single 12 lead ECG which may be normal is worthless in ruling out acute myocardial infarction, since changes may never appear or may be delayed for hours. Careful studies of serial ECGs should be obtained and correlated with other findings. It is important to appreciate that myocardial infarction may be found at autopsy, and the patient may never have had a diagnosis of infarction made during life.

The infarction process progresses through three phases:

1. Hyperacute phase
2. Fully evolved phase
3. Phase of resolution

Hyperacute phase

This occurs within the first hours of the onset of acute myocardial infarction. The transition from this to the fully evolved phase usually occurs within 24 hours, and so it is frequently missed.

The ST segment is elevated and there is a tall and widened T wave (at times exceeding the height of the R wave). The *pathological* Q wave does not occur until this large T wave has regressed. There is also increased ventricular activation time, i.e. the time from the beginning of the QRS complex to the apex of the R wave (see Fig. 30).

Fully evolved phase

Myocardial necrosis is reflected by a broad deep Q wave (pathological Q wave) in electrodes facing the necrotic area.

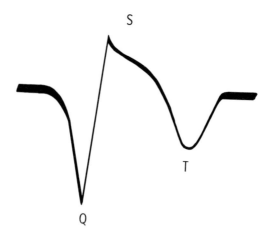

Fig. 57. *Typical infarction pattern: deep Q wave, raised and coved ST segment and inverted T wave.*

Dead tissue is electrically inert and therefore it cannot be activated or depolarized. If there is a transmural infarct, this can be described electrically as a 'window' or 'hole' in the muscle wall. An electrode placed over this 'window' reflects activity of other muscle as 'seen' through this 'window'. If an electrode is placed over an area of dead muscle in the left ventricular wall, depolarization occurs as usual, from the left side of the septum to the right. Thus a small negative deflection will be inscribed on the ECG. Subsequently depolarization spreads to affect the right ventricle, resulting in a further negative deflection on the ECG. This results in the pathological Q wave of myocardial infarction. Pathological Q waves are wide (0.04 s or longer in duration), deep (usually greater than 4 mm in depth), usually associated with a substantial loss in the height of the ensuing R wave, and usually present in several leads. It is important to note that a Q wave in lead III is frequently present normally. This 'normal' Q wave usually diminishes or disappears on deep inspiration, whereas the 'pathological' Q wave persists. Normally, Q waves are also present in leads facing the left ventricle and in AVR. They are also commonly found in V1 and V2. Pathological Q waves usually persist indefinitely because the scar tissue which replaces the infarcted muscle is similarly uninvolved in electrical activation.

Myocardial injury is reflected by displacement of the ST segment.

Myocardial injury in most infarctions is dominantly epicardial, and this is present on the ECG with elevated ST segments in the leads facing this surface. The ST segment in the fully evolved phase of the infarction is coved (or convex-upward). The exact mechanism of these ST segment shifts is controversial.

Myocardial ischaemia is reflected by an inverted T wave.

T wave inversion occurs in those leads facing the ischaemic surface. They are characteristically 'arrowhead' in appearance being peaked and symmetrical.

An infarcted area consists of necrotic tissue surrounded by a zone of injured tissue which is in turn surrounded by a zone of ischaemic tissue. The *typical infarct pattern* consists of the pathological Q wave, the raised coved ST segment, and the inverted, pointed symmetrical T wave.

Phase of resolution

This phase follows on from the fully evolved phase. During the following weeks, there is a gradual return of the elevated ST segment to the baseline. The inverted symmetrical T waves gradually return to a normal or near-normal configuration, but they may persist for months. The only evidence of a myocardial infarction may be a pathological Q wave.

If ST segment elevation persists after six months, a ventricular aneurysm should be suspected.

LOCATION OF MYOCARDIAL INFARCTION

As already stated, infarcts occur predominantly in the anterior, inferior, and posterior walls of the left ventricle.

Anterior infarction

The anterior surface of the left ventricle is orientated towards the chest leads. The anterolateral surface of the left ventricle is orientated towards lead AVL and the positive pole of standard lead I. Thus anterior infarcts will be reflected by the typical infarct pattern (pathological Q waves, raised ST segments, and inverted T waves) in leads I, AVL and the chest leads (V1, 2, 3, 4, 5, and 6).

Anterior infarcts can be sub-divided into:

Extensive anterior infarction: Infarct pattern in leads I, AVL and V1 - V6.

Anteroseptal infarction: Infarct pattern in leads V1 - V4.

Anterolateral infarction: Infarct pattern in leads I, AVL and V4 - V6.

Inferior infarction

The inferior surface of the left ventricle is orientated towards standard leads II, III, and AVF. Thus, inferior infarcts will be reflected by the typical infarct pattern in leads II, III, and AVF.

Posterior infarction

True posterior infarction is uncommon. The typical infarct pattern of the ECG does not occur, because none of the leads are orientated towards the true posterior surface of the heart. Therefore, the diagnosis is made from 'inverse' changes in leads which are orientated towards the uninjured (anterior) surface of the heart: leads V1 and V2. These leads show tall and slightly widened R waves; tall, wide and symmetrical T waves; and slightly depressed, *concave*-upward ST segments. The combination of these changes in the right chest leads occurring in true posterior infarction is the 'mirror-image' of the typical infarct pattern which would be recorded by a lead orientated towards the true posterior wall.

Further ECG leads may be required for infarcts in unusual sites. In high anterior and lateral infarcts, V7 and V8 and leads recorded in the second or third intercostal space may be useful.

The recognition of acute myocardial infarction on the ECG may be difficult if there has been previous infarction which has resulted in persistent Q waves, ST segment elevation, or T wave inversion. Left bundle branch block may confuse the situation.

Subendocardial infarction

A subendocardial infarction may cause ST segment depression and T wave inversion. However, pathological Q waves are absent.

INFARCT SIZE DETERMINATION

Considerable research has been done in an effort to measure the size of infarction and to develop methods of decreasing the size of the infarcted area. This is generally based on three principles:

1. The mass of damaged myocardium determines the prognosis.
2. The mass of damaged myocardium can be measured quantitatively.
3. The damaged myocardium may be modified by appropriate treatment.

A number of techniques have been used to determine the extent and evolution of myocardial ischaemia. These include:

1. ST segment analysis of the ECG.
2. Creatine phosphokinase (CPK) changes.
3. Nuclear imaging.

ENZYMES

Necrosis of the myocardium results in the release of the enzymes normally contained within it. Large quantities of the enzymes are released into the circulation which are then detectable by laboratory investigation. The rate of liberation of specific enzymes differs following infarction, and the pattern of enzyme release is therefore important. Serial enzyme studies are pointless if the suspected infarction occurred more than a few days before a blood sample is taken.

Creatine phosphokinase (CPK)

This is found mainly in heart, skeletal muscle and brain. It consists of two sub-units, each of which may be either type B (occurring mainly in brain) or type M (occurring mainly in muscle). Thus three isoenzymes may be formed: CPK-MM, CPK-BB, and CPK-MB. The latter is virtually specific for cardiac muscle. CPK is usually raised 6 hours after infarction, reaching a peak in 18 – 24 hours. It declines rapidly, reaching basal levels two to four days after infarction.

It is important to appreciate that a two to three-fold elevation of CPK may follow an intra-muscular injection. This may lead to the false diagnosis of acute myocardial infarction in a patient who has been given an IM injection of an analgesic for chest pain of non-cardiac origin.

Other potential sources of CPK elevation include muscle diseases, hypothyroidism, and stroke. By contrast, CPK-MB is unaffected in these circumstances.

Myoglobin (MG)

This has recently been used in the diagnosis of acute myocardial infarction. It appears in the blood stream before CPK and is also eliminated faster.

Aspartate aminotransferase (ASAT or AAT)

Glutamic oxaloacetic transaminase (GOT) is now commonly known as ASAT. It is found particularly in heart, skeletal muscle, brain, liver, and kidney. Following acute myocardial infarction the increase in ASAT starts at about the same time as that of CPK, reaching a peak in 24 – 36 hours, returning to normal from about the third day.

Alanine aminotransferase (ALAT)

Glutamic pyruvate transaminase (GPT) is now commonly known as ALAT. It is abundant in the liver but sparse in the myocardium. The time course is slightly retarded in comparison to that of ASAT.

Lactic dehydrogenase (LDH)

This is found in heart, skeletal muscle, brain, liver, kidney, and erythrocytes. It has five isoenzymes which can be separated and occur in varying proportions in each tissue. The LDH_1 and LDH_2 isoenzymes are the myocardial fraction that rises after myocardial infarction. LDH rises relatively late after infarction and reaches a peak at 24 – 48 hours. Increased activity is maintained during at least one week thereafter.

Alpha-hydroxybutyric dehydrogenase (HBD)

Some laboratories routinely measure HBD as an indirect measure of LDH_1 and LDH_2.

Diagnostic ranges of each enzyme test will vary from one laboratory to another.

In most cases routine enzyme measurement with the use of CPK, ASAT and LDH/HBD helps to decide the diagnosis.

The clinical picture, serial ECGs and serial enzyme levels are usually sufficient to establish the diagnosis of myocardial infarction.

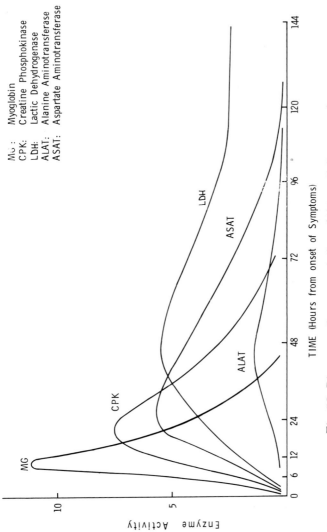

Mʊ :   Myoglobin
CPK: Creatine Phosphokinase
LDH: Lactic Dehydrogenase
ALAT: Alanine Aminotransferase
ASAT: Aspartate Aminotransferase

Fig. 58. *Diagrammatic representation of time-activity curves for diagnostic enzymes following acute myocardial infarction.*

CORONARY CARE

INTRODUCTION

The World Health Organization (WHO) in a recent report (1979) drew attention to the concept of *comprehensive cardiac care*. In the context of an acute myocardial infarction this comprises of pre-hospital prophylaxis with community involvement and early management, coronary care in hospital (in a specialized unit or general ward), and post-hospital care with progressive rehabilitation and secondary prevention.

AIMS OF CORONARY CARE UNITS

It was recognized that the commonest cause of early death after acute myocardial infarction was ventricular fibrillation (VF), and the development of DC countershock meant that by prompt intervention, an otherwise fatal arrhythmia could be corrected. This led to the creation of coronary care units (CCUs) where the original aim was to detect VF and to use a prepared programme for resuscitation from this arrhythmia. These units were established in the early 1960s in the USA, Australia, Canada and the UK, where it was indicated that the provision of such units was mandatory for patients with myocardial infarction. It was generally accepted that the CCU led to a reduction in the hospital mortality rate of patients with acute myocardial infarction.

In the past decade, CCUs have become widespread in the UK, yet there has been no reduction in the overall mortality from infarcts, the observed fall in hospital mortality possibly resulting from an increase in admissions of low-risk cases rather than the efficacy of CCUs.

Continuous ECG monitoring on these units revealed that serious cardiac arrhythmias were much more common than had been appreciated previously, and that they often gave warning of the onset of ventricular tachycardia/fibrillation and asystole. Therefore, attention has been directed towards the prevention of cardiac arrest and to the earlier detection and treatment of lesser, warning arrhythmias.

No adequate randomized trial of the long-term value of intensive coronary care has yet been carried out. It has to be admitted that the therapeutic potential of the CCU is limited and that the practical management of patients with acute coronary episodes has not dramatically changed, in spite of a tremendous amount of research. However, the principle of coronary care is still to provide first class resuscitation facilities in a peaceful and reassuring atmosphere. It is extremely doubtful that a patient developing VF would stand the same chance of survival as in a CCU.

It has often been stated that the journey to hospital and the strange environment in which the patient is placed, offset the benefits of hospital care. A very high proportion of acute coronary deaths (mainly VF)—about 50%—occurs in the first hour. Under these circumstances many deaths will occur in the ambulance. Yet there is little evidence to suggest that a journey in a modern ambulance, itself contributes to the mortality. There is generally a widespread fear of hospital in the community, and more so of CCUs; yet the patient can be reasonably assured that the CCU is a place for getting better under observation. Realizing that the patient's fears are both normal and understandable responses to hospitalization, the health team, and particularly the nurse, should recognize their duty to establish an effective communications link with the patient at this crucial time, even though to do so may be a quite trying task.

The CCU is an excellent place for the nurse to begin a rehabilitation programme: the patient can be encouraged to stop smoking, reduce weight, and start progressive exercises with a view to returning to work. He can nearly always be told truthfully that a rapid recovery is expected.

CORONARY CARE VERSUS HOME CARE

Recently there have been increasing arguments for home care as opposed to coronary care for patients with acute myocardial infarction. Critics state that the CCUs can themselves give rise to problems by frightening patients, that they have not been proven to be effective and that they are expensive to run.

Studies have been carried out in which patients have been randomly allocated to home or hospital care. Results showed that there was no statistical difference in the mortality of these patients in the two places of management. Although these studies were criticised, they did however point out that some patients may be better managed at home, and that the beneficial effects of intensive coronary care are probably confined to patients seen within the first few hours or to those with complications. (*Mather et al 1971; Hill et al 1978*)

The major question to be answered is not whether patients with coronary attacks should be managed at home or in hospital, but how the early high mortality from VF can be reduced. Reduction in delay

between the onset of symptoms and the call for help is clearly impera-
tive. In order that this delay is reduced to a minimum, constant education of the public regarding the symptoms of the coronary attack is
essential. Education of the public about initiating cardiopulmonary
resuscitation would undoubtedly save more lives. The only area which
practices this technique is the Seattle system in the USA, which uses
trained paramedical personnel to resuscitate patients from VF outside
hospital.

Home care
There are certainly some patients who are obviously better off at
home. These include:

(a) Patients over 60 years of age; especially if there is no hypo-
    tension, heart failure, or persistence of pain.
(b) Patients seen some time after the presumed onset of the attack,
    provided the attack is uncomplicated.
(c) The patient's home is some distance from a hospital, especially
    if this has no intensive care facilities.
(d) Patients wish to have home care.

If the patient's doctor is called at all, the symptoms will probably
have lasted for a long time and the patient will already have survived
the period of greatest risk of a dangerous arrhythmia before receiving
medical help. However, there is still a risk of unexpected problems in
this group.

The GP should be familiar with modern coronary care practice and
in the use of a defibrillator and monitor. Many GPs do not have ECG
machines, and are unused to reading the tracings. The two hours
needed to control the acute problems and get the patient 'stabilized'
could probably take the same approach as a group in Nottingham.
There, a mobile team consisting of a junior doctor and CCU trained
nurse, go to the patient's home in response to calls from GPs about
patients with suspected infarcts. The teams most important clinical
role was to ensure adequate pain relief. A two-hour wait under observation allowed safer transfer to hospital if this was needed on social
grounds or if there were signs of impending problems.

Mobile coronary care units
Mobile coronary care units (MCCUs) were pioneered in 1966 in Belfast

to enable personnel trained in coronary care to reach the patient at the site of the coronary attack (at home or elsewhere) as soon as possible after the onset of symptoms. The MCCU is manned by a doctor and a nurse, and is always on 'stand-by'. GPs can reach the CCU directly by means of a special telephone number. A short-wave radio system enables the duty doctor to receive immediately the call for the MCCU. These units have proved very successful; resuscitating 10 – 40% of patients from VF outside hospital. Unfortunately, there are only a handful of these units in the UK.

THE NURSING ROLE IN THE CORONARY CARE SYSTEM

The nurse is the key to the entire programme in the coronary care system. The term system is used to encompass hospital (CCU) and home care of the coronary patient. The nurse's main commitment is to nursing care, while providing clinical leadership, defining the nursing needs of the patient, and identifying and analysing nursing problems and priorities. The nurse must seek solutions to these problems and administer and provide effective care.

The nurse's responsibilities can be categorized as follows:

1. To share with the physician the responsibility for patient care.
2. To identify systematically the nursing needs of patients.
3. To devise and implement appropriate nursing care plans for individual patients.
4. To carry her own case load.
5. To make observations of patients' needs and evaluate nursing requirements.
6. To coordinate procedures, tests, and personnel for the patients for whom she is responsible.
7. To translate research findings into actual nursing practice.
8. To institute improvements in patient care.
9. To initiate preventive measures to protect the patient from complications.
10. To serve as a model of expert clinical nursing.

The nurse is responsible for controlling and manipulating the patient's environment so as to promote his well being and comfort while carrying out the established objectives of care simultaneously. (*Abdellah 1972*)

On the CCU the nurse has more opportunity to observe the patient continuously than any other member of the health team. To enable her to observe the patients in a meaningful way, it is necessary for her to have special technical knowledge appropriate to the needs of the patients in her care.

Continuity of care is generally acknowledged by nurses as well as others in the health team as an essential component of health care. Unfortunately, the consistency with which it is rendered remains less than satisfactory in too many instances.

The focus of care in the CCU is centred primarily on the prevention of complications rather than dealing with them as they occur. The nurse plays a unique role in health education, prevention and rehabilitation, and these will be discussed later. The nurse must also assume responsibility for decision-making. She will need to formulate and implement nursing policies, and establish effective working relationships with other members of the health team.

Primary health care

The nurse is and will increasingly assume more responsibility as a member of the primary health care team. The role of the nurse in the acute phases of the illness may be either contributory or supportive. She acquires further skill in obtaining and evaluating a health history, interpreting selected diagnostic tests, health teaching and health counselling.

ADMISSION TO THE CORONARY CARE UNIT

The nurse who cares for the patient immediately upon admission may greatly influence the patient's subsequent course of recovery. The behaviour, attitudes and nursing skills of the nurse during the patient's initial response to this stressful situation may mean the difference between success and failure in the patient's eventual rehabilitation. Possibly the morale of the nursing staff and others on the CCU is the single most important determinant of patient satisfaction.

It is well to introduce the patient (and his family) to the members of staff, explain the need for his hospitalization, various tests, and how long he is likely to remain on the unit. It is reassuring to explain that he can be expected to mobilize rapidly and that there is no reason why he should not be able to leave hospital after about eight days, providing no complications occur. It is important to include the family in all future plans regarding rehabilitation. During the admission procedure the family will probably be asked to wait in another area, but they should be assured that the wait will be short, that someone will come to talk to them, and that they will be allowed to visit the patient once he has been admitted. This approach will help the nurse to assess more thoroughly all aspects of the patient in order to plan appropriate patient care.

Observation

Two primary and essential functions of the nurse in observing the patient are 'to look' and 'to listen'. The art of quick and accurate observation is a highly cultivated skill. Heart rate and rhythm, skin appearance, chest movements, and psychological state can be observed quickly and unobtrusively even before monitor recordings are made. It is important to remember that the patient is more important than the monitor.

Monitoring

Most patients accept being attached to a monitor, indeed, they often feel more secure because of this. However, they do tend to object or feel anxious about the alarm buzzer. The nurse should explain about the monitor's function in positive terms emphasizing its routine use with coronary patients and that it signifies the presence of no special trouble. This often diminishes whatever unresolved fears the patient may have. It is important to describe erratic patterns in their ECG and explain that they are unrelated to heart activity, but caused by position change and movement.

It seems strange, but patients tend to put their trust in machines with great ease. In working with cardiac monitors, the nurse should understand their purpose, limitations and problems. None of them are perfect and trouble-free.

Most coronary care units have a central monitoring console at the nurse's station. These are usually equipped with rhythm strip print-outs that may be worked manually or automatically to obtain an ECG print-out of the patient. Memory loops, which record and store for a specific period of time each patient's ECG rhythm, are also usually available. This magnetic tape recording system can be activated automatically to hold and not erase the ECG of the 10 s to 5 min preceding the incident.

All the systems for acquiring and monitoring the ECG are designed around a few basic elements: sensors, transmission links, and processing devices. The sensors are the skin electrodes placed on either the chest or limbs. Chest electrodes are preferred, because a clearer signal can be obtained with a better definition of the smaller ECG deflections such as the P wave. Transmission takes place along wires, although radio-telemetry is now very popular. Processing requires amplification of the signal after which it may be displayed on an oscilloscope, a paper chart recorder, or recorded on to magnetic tape for analysis later. If computer facilities are available, an automatic analysis and interpretation can be provided.

The design and performance of the electrode is important. Features that need to be considered by the nurse are:

1. The ease and speed of application
2. The ability to produce a clear ECG trace
3. The cost

Most electrodes are pre-gelled and disposable. The patient's chest needs to be cleaned, and any hair shaved to prevent irritation and interference with conduction. The electrodes are then placed on the desired site and then attached to lead wires. A clear ECG pattern should then be obtained. The longer the electrode is in use the more likely are skin reactions to develop.

Electrocardiographic monitoring commonly requires three chest electrodes. These are usually placed on the two infraclavicular areas and over the right sternal edge, away from large muscle masses, therefore minimizing muscle artifact. It is preferable to use a modified lead V1 (MCL – I), as advocated by Marriott (1970), in which the negative electrode is on the left shoulder; the positive electrode is at the right sternal edge in the fourth intercostal space; and the ground electrode is on the right shoulder. This lead configuration generally demonstrates good amplitude P waves and allows detection of left and right bundle branch block and the distinction of left ventricular ectopic beats from supraventricular impulses conducted with right bundle branch aberration.

It is the practice of most coronary care units to obtain a standard 12-lead ECG immediately upon admission to the unit and routinely every morning during the patient's stay in the unit. Additional 12-lead ECGs are obtained any time the patient complains of a new onset of chest pain or when changes are noted on the monitor suggesting alterations in intra-ventricular conduction.

GENERAL PRINCIPLES OF PATIENT CARE

The principles of patient care are to relieve symptoms (pain and anxiety), prevent their recurrence, promote healing (rest), and prevent complications. Obviously care plans will be developed individually, depending on the physiological and psychological responses to myocardial infarction in each patient. However, these principles provide a framework to build upon.

Rest

Nowadays, patients with an uncomplicated myocardial infarction are kept in bed for 24 - 48 hours only. Thereafter, gradual mobilization should encourage them to walk around the ward by the end of a few days. Although the patient is placed on bed rest for the first day or two, he should be allowed to 'self-care', unless the activities he performs are increasing metabolic activity to an undesirable level. The patient's pulse and blood pressure are excellent measurements for judging this. Self-care activities which should be allowed include washing, eating, and shaving. For too long, nurses have been insisting on carrying out these 'duties', supposedly for the 'patient's benefit'. Clearly, each patient's individual needs are assessed separately by the nurse responsible for administering that patient's care. Care plans, therefore, need to be developed and evaluated so that patient care is consistent. For many patients the stress of not being allowed any degree of independence in self-care activities causes more energy expenditure than the performance of the actual activity would. It is important to stress that only nursing care that is essential to the patient's well-being and comfort be carried out. For too long, nurses have been carrying out rituals and routines without justifying them to be truly in the best interest of patient care.

Rest periods should be provided during the day, for although the CCU should ideally be an environment for resting, it is usually far from being so. Sensory deprivation and unnecessary noise are frequently experienced by these patients. The noise and unnecessary activity should be kept to the minimum. This does not mean that the patient should be isolated and discouraged from conversing with staff and fellow patients. Indeed, the environment should be stimulating and warm. The nurse should engage the patient in psychological and physiological stimulation, as boredom is a common problem which frequently results from enforced bed-rest. This can often precipitate mood changes, namely anxiety and depression, and the nurse should be alert for these. The patient's family have much to offer in allaying these problems, and need to be actively involved in the care and rehabilitation of the patients. Visiting from family members, particularly the spouse, should be encouraged, and not frowned upon. Visitors are frequently viewed with suspicion, as if they pose a threat to the nurse-patient relationship. Yet this should not be so, and families should be seen as allies, not distractions or obstacles to care. Clearly, visiting arrangements will depend on various factors. However, visiting should be relatively flexible and open-ended for family members or close friends. The provision of clocks, radios, newspapers, television, and personal items such as photographs, can do much to assist the patient in preventing sensory deprivation.

During the first 24 hours, the patient should be encouraged to carry out deep breathing and relaxation exercises. Following this period, some patients will be allowed up in a chair, either for bed making or for an hour or so. This early mobilization is a sign of progress to the patient and improves his morale. Also, the cardiac workload is lighter when the patient is in a sitting position rather than a reclining position. If no untoward effects occur, the patient is allowed to sit in the chair for longer periods, according to his tolerance. The patient should also be asked to report any symptoms which may indicate over-exertion. These include chest pain, shortness of breath, palpitations, syncope. Although gradual mobilization should be encouraged it is important to avoid undue fatigue. The patient may over-exert, and the need for temporary limitation must be stressed, In uncomplicated cases the patient may walk freely towards the end of the first week. In complicated cases mobilization should be slightly slower. Most patients can be fully mobilized within 7 - 10 days, after which time they should be allowed (if able) to climb the stairs in the hospital before they are sent home.

Bed rest, even for 24 hours, can lead to many hazards, and nursing intervention should be aimed at preventing them. Once the pain has subsided, patients should be encouraged to move their feet and legs to minimize the risk of thrombophlebitis.

Other problems associated with immobility are dealt with as follows.

Bowels

Prolonged bed rest decreases gastrointestinal activity, and the faeces may become hardened because of water reabsorption. Straining and attempts to use a bedpan should be avoided because they may result in excessive isometric work, which is undesirable because it serves as a vagal stimulant which may produce bradycardia and provoke other arrhythmias. Therefore, a bedside commode is recommended. Patients should be reassured that it will not be harmful to go without a bowel movement for several days, but if the patient is distressed and uncomfortable, a laxative may be given.

Urine output

Another problem associated with prolonged bed rest is difficult in urinating. An adequate fluid intake is usually all that is required to alleviate this. The patient should be encouraged to void frequently, but to avoid unnecessary stress. A male patient may experience difficulty in voiding in a supine position, and the nurse must be aware that certain drugs (e.g. disopyramide) may cause urinary retention. If possible, the patient should be allowed to stand out of bed, in order to make voiding easier. It is important to appreciate that the patient needs privacy; a male member of staff, if available, should stay with the patient.

Pain

The relief of pain is one of the most important objectives of patient care. The nurse needs to assess the pain by obtaining the patient's own description of it and observing the individual's reaction to it. Before nurses actually decide what intervention is indicated, it is always wise to consider whether any bias has limited their ability to assess the patient's needs correctly. For example, nurses who believe that patients should stand some pain before taking a drug tend to believe that these patients tolerate pain well.

Apart from reducing pain, fear and distress, an opiate will reduce catecholamine release which may decrease the tendency to ventricular arrhythmias. Their vasodilator effects will reduce afterload and could conceivably reduce infarct size and improve heart failure.

Diamorphine or morphine are the drugs of choice, although their depressant effects on the respiratory centre need to be remembered. They should preferably be given intravenously, both to achieve rapid action and to avoid localized muscle damage with enzyme release. The intramuscular injection of many drugs results in release of creatine phosphokinase (CPK) which may interfere with the subsequent laboratory diagnosis of the infarction. They should be given in quite large doses initially. Those patients with bradycardia should be given atropine with or before the opiate. Pethidine and pentazocine have adverse haemodynamic effects, and are therefore not particularly desirable. Diamorphine (heroin) is about 2.5 times more potent than morphine as an analgesic.

Sedation

This is an important problem in the CCU, where the general atmosphere of 24 hour observation may interfere with the patient's sleep. Most patients require sedation to withstand better the period of enforced inactivity (bed-rest). A mild tranquillizer, such as diazepam (Valium) lessens anxiety and produces mild sedation. The patient may also require chlormethiazole (Heminevrin) or nitrazepam (Mogadon) at night time.

It must be remembered that sedation is no substitute for a dark, quiet environment.

Oxygen

Most patients with acute myocardial infarction have a reduced arterial PO_2. The routine use of oxygen is based on the assumption that it increases the PO_2 of the blood and therefore becomes responsible for the diffusion of oxygen into the ischaemic myocardium. However, there appears to be no evidence of benefit from this practice although there is none of harm either. Oxygen should be administered in severely ill patients with left ventricular failure, hypotension or cardiogenic shock. The usual method of administration is by means of a nasal catheter or a face mask at a flow of 4 – 8 litres per minute, which results in an oxygen concentration of 28 – 35%.

Oxygen should always be humidified when it is administered, and mouth and nose care should be given. The skin should also be checked for pressure marks.

Anticoagulant therapy

The use of anticoagulants in the management of patients with acute myocardial infarction is a controversial issue. It does seem to reduce the incidence of deep vein thrombosis, and pulmonary and systemic emboli; however with early mobilization, deep vein thrombosis and pulmonary embolism are relatively uncommon. Although the evidence is confused, a few believe there is sufficient reason to give anticoagulants for up to one year after infarction in order to prevent pulmonary embolism, and to prevent further myocardial infarction. In patients with atrial fibrillation, there is stasis in the ineffectively contracting atrium which encourages thrombosis. Because the risk of embolism is particularly high, heparin should be given.

Heparin can be given in the form of:

(a) *A continuous infusion:* A loading dose of 5000 - 10 000 units is given, followed by 15 000 units 12 hourly. It is important to give heparin in a normal saline infusion rather than Dextrose which can unpredictably reduce the anticoagulant effect.

(b) *Intermittent intravenous therapy:* This can be given as 10 000 units six hourly.

(c) *Low dose subcutaneous heparin:* This is used prophylactically to prevent deep vein thrombosis. For example, 'Mini-dose Heparin', 5 000 units 12 hourly.

Oral anticoagulants are often begun in conjunction with heparin. The usual loading dose for warfarin is 10 – 30 mg. The effect is monitored by measuring the prothrombin time 48 hours later when maintenance doses are started according to this. There is little evidence that abrupt cessation of oral anticoagulant therapy results in a rebound hyper-coaguable state. It is therefore unnecessary to taper off the dose. The long half-life of oral anticoagulants ensures that a sudden cessation of dosage does not mean a sudden fall in the plasma drug level.

PSYCHOLOGICAL ASPECTS

The first and most important aspect of patient care is the recognition of any anxiety or fear that the patient might be experiencing. This may be handled well by building a relationship within the framework of reassurance. The nurse should listen to the patient in a calm, unhurried, and sympathetic and empathetic manner. She should establish a mutual relationship of trust, thus providing a therapeutic environment for the patient in which both psychological and physical needs can be met. Primary nursing is the ideal method of patient care. In this way, contact between the nurse and patient is at its best.

The psychological reactions of patients to their infarct vary with the individual. Fear of death is inherent in many of these patients, although during the acute phase of the illness the stress is generally physical. Psychological stress begins in the recovery phase. Following discharge, many patients undergo an identity crisis. The nurse can help the patient to accept his illness by group identity and introduction to other patients who have had similar experiences.

Nursing intervention needs to be aimed at recognizing the patient's manifestations of psychological stress, helping the patient to recognize them, and helping him cope with them. The nurse can do much to reduce the stress of the coronary care environment by appropriate communication. Recent research by *Ashworth* (*1980*) has highlighted some of the problems and deficiencies of communication between patients and nurses.

Coping mechanisms
The principle coping mechanism here is denial. It is interesting to note that denial seems to be a valuable defence mechanism in terms of reducing mortality and morbidity in the CCU. Here, the nurse can reassure these patients by emphasizing their good prognosis, when this is realistic.

Mood changes
The most common mood changes experienced by the patient are anxiety and depression. The depression is usually reactive in nature. Information given in a positive and encouraging manner, and the use of adequate night sedation can often allay these mood changes. What is needed is sensitivity, listening, and awareness on the part of the nurse and the appropriate reaction to the individual patient's mood/situation, etc.

Patients witnessing a cardiac arrest
Apart from suffering a cardiac arrest oneself, witnessing one is the most stressful of all experiences in the CCU. Even though the event may be unseen, patients can hear and (usually incorrectly) imagine what is happening.

Surviving a cardiac arrest
The majority of patients who experience a cardiac arrest are unable to recall much of the event. It appears that with the passage of time, unless recently reminded, the patient forgets what happened. However, patients who have sustained multiple arrests can often recall cardiac massage prior to losing consciousness and also the pain of having a shock pass through the chest wall.

Stress on the nurse
One of the most impressive features of the CCU is the competence of the nursing staff. However, recurring stressful situations are not uncommon,

e.g. staff friction, responding to a cardiac arrest, and dealing with a patient's death. Nurses tend to choose to work in CCU *because* it proceeds at a hectic pace, under high tension and caring for very ill patients.

There are ways of coping with the stresses of CCU, and these include regular group meetings, adequate staffing levels, and adequate meal breaks. (*Cassem and Hackett 1975*)

Weekly group meetings are a useful way of dealing with stress on the nurse. She can identify, acknowledge, and share her feelings with the group who can then review their own experiences with criticism, support, and praise. In order for successful group encounters, the place of the meetings needs to be accessible, where nurses (and other unit members) can feel free to come and go at any moment. The group will need a facilitator who knows what is going on. Any member of staff who possesses the required skills should be able to facilitate.

NURSING STAFF PROBLEMS IN THE CCU

Nurses working in the CCU have tended to have certain psychological characteristics. Studies have shown that they tend to score higher on indices of depression, hostility, and anxiety than nurses who work in general medical wards. This probably stems, in part, from heavy work loads, increased responsibility, confined working area, and inadequate continuing education programmes. (*Cassem and Hackett 1975*)

Self-esteem can be easily damaged by 'being singled out' to help on a general ward. A rota where this is shared equally can prevent these feelings. Nurses from other areas may accuse the coronary care nurse as being over-rated and under-worked. However, if the coronary care nurse feels competent and secure, less friction is generated. Excessive competition is a most disruptive element in the CCU, i.e. the nurse who wants to 'be in charge'. Scapegoating is another major problem. Efficiency and tidiness are convenient to indicate that one is angry or upset about something. These nurses tend to feel that they are the only ones who care about 'their patients' on the unit. Scapegoating of the charge nurse or Nursing Officer is very common. These people are expected to be super-efficient.

If all staff members are allowed active participation and given recognition and respect for their opinions, interpersonal relationships and morale will be greatly improved.

TRANSFER FROM THE CORONARY CARE UNIT

Transfer from the CCU usually occurs two to three days after infarction or when monitoring is no longer a high priority. Patients may feel anxious about transfer from the CCU even when it is discussed with them beforehand. Although transfer is generally viewed by the patient to be evidence of progress, increased anxiety is not unusual. The sudden disruption of a high nurse-patient ratio, new staff and unfamiliar environment can cause exacerbation of an illness, and it is not uncommon for these patients to have arrhythmias and extension of the infarct soon after transfer to the ward. In most CCUs the nursing staff tend to focus on the 'here and now' and give little thought in preparing the patient for eventual transfer.

It is important to make the transition from the CCU to the ward as smooth as possible. The nurse who has had most contact with the patient and his family should assist in the transfer. The patient should be introduced to the ward staff and, if possible, be placed in a bed close to the nurses' station. It would be helpful if the nurse from the ward met the patient on CCU prior to the actual transfer, thus allaying any fears. It is important that a thorough report and assessment of the patient should accompany him. The patient's family should be informed of the transfer, either by the patient or the nurse who has been caring for him.

COMPLICATIONS OF ACUTE MYOCARDIAL INFARCTION

Arrhythmias

These are an almost universal accompaniment of acute myocardial infarction. Some, such as asystole and VF are of obvious importance because they carry a high mortality.

Sinus bradycardia. This is seen in about 15% of all patients and is more common immediately after infarction and in patients with inferior infarction. It is usually harmless, but if it produces hypotension or is associated with ventricular ectopic activity, atropine 0.3 mg IV should be given and repeated if necessary. If the bradycardia does not respond to this, then use of a temporary transvenous pacemaker may be indicated.

Supraventricular arrhythmias. Atrial tachycardia, flutter and fibrillation occur in about 20% of patients; they are often transient, being secondary to left ventricular failure. Rapid ventricular rates should be treated with anti-arrhythmic therapy (e.g. Digoxin, Oubaine, Verapamil or Practolol, IV). If the arrhythmia persists with a critical haemodynamic deterioration cardioversion should be carried out. Junctional arrhythmias are usually of little clinical importance.

Ventricular ectopic beats. These occur in almost all patients with acute myocardial infarction. This incidence and the fact that VF can arise as a result of a single VEB, has led to much intensive research. VEBs are dangerous if:

   (a) they are of 'R on T' variety
   (b) multifocal
   (c) frequently, or consecutively occurring

These types are often precursors of ventricular tachycardia (VT) or VF. Anti-arrhythmic therapy should be given to suppress VEBs. Lignocaine is the treatment of choice because it acts rapidly and its effects disappear soon (15 - 20 minutes) after its administration is discontinued. Lignocaine is given initially as a single IV injection (bolus) of 50 - 100 mg to establish adequate blood levels quickly. This should be followed by an infusion of 1 - 2 mg per minute. Usually, VEBs spontaneously disappear after about 72 hours.

Ventricular tachycardia. This is associated with a high mortality, because it can cause haemodynamic deterioration and lead to VF. It appears that VT is associated with a worsened prognosis only when it occurs at rates above 140 per minute. Sustained VT is usually treated primarily with Lignocaine. Oral anti-arrhythmic therapy (e.g. Procainamide or Mexiletine) is usually started when intravenous therapy is stopped. If VT cannot be terminated by these means, cardioversion should be used.

Ventricular fibrillation. This is the usual cause of sudden death, which is most common within the first hour following acute myocardial infarction. The long-term survival is good in patients with *primary* VF (VF resulting as a primary response to acute ischaemia and not associated with predisposing factors such as heart failure or cardiogenic shock). Another form, *secondary* VF, complicates the course of patients with heart failure and/or hypotension, and considerably worsens the prognosis (which is in any case bad). Cardioversion (defibrillation or DC shock) is used immediately in patients with VF. The improvement of oxygenation and perfusion and the correction of acidosis increases the likelihood of successful defibrillation. Bretylium is a drug that is effective against VF refractory to Lignocaine and multiple DC shock, but does not seem to be commonly used. A new anti-arrhythmic drug, amiodarone (Cordarone X), when given intravenously has shown that it is rapidly effective for supraventricular tachycardia, ventricular ectopic beats, ventricular tachycardia, and ventricular fibrillation.

It is pertinent to discuss the role of the nurse in dealing with these rhythm disturbances. Because the nurse is the person most frequently encountered by the patient, she is often expected to urgently deal with life-threatening situations; most obviously VF, before medical help arrives. The nurse needs to be fully competent at dealing with these emergencies, and the coronary care nurse is expected to carry out many procedures not normally performed by other nurses. These procedures include:

Cardioversion
Venous cannulation
Setting up a drip

Before continuing to outline further complications of acute myocardial infarction, these three procedures will be covered in some depth.

CARDIOVERSION

Cardioversion or direct current (DC) shock therapy is a method of terminating arrhythmias, by means of externally applied, electrical shock.

THEORY

When an ectopic disorder is momentarily extinguished, the sinus node, which has the highest rhythmicity in the heart, resumes as the dominant pacemaker. The heart can be depolarised across the chest by electrical discharge. When effective, such depolarization abolishes the ectopic mechanism and permits restoration of sinus rhythm.

Direct current (DC) shock therapy may be used to defibrillate the heart. This is more effective in depolarizing the heart, induces fewer arrhythmias and less tissue damage than alternating current (AC) shock. The only hazard associated with this therapy is the sporadic occurrence of ventricular fibrillation (VF).

When the DC discharge is delivered systematically through the cardiac cycle, VF occurs only when the discharge is triggered during the final one-third of systole. This vulnerable period has a duration of 30 m.s and just precedes the upstroke of the T wave of the ECG. When a DC discharge is triggered outside this period VF does not occur. Thus by synchronizing the release of the discharge within a safe part of the cardiac cycle, that is, 30 m.s *after* the beginning of the QRS complex, VF (and ventricular standstill) can be avoided.

This technique (cardioversion) is used for terminating a diversity of ectopic arrhythmias which have not responded to drug therapy.

It is important to note that nurses only carry out cardioversion as an *emergency* procedure (i.e. for termination of VT/VF), and not as an *elective procedure.*

TECHNIQUE

This procedure is essentially the same irrespective of the type of arrhythmia. If the procedure is elective, it is explained to the patient. A consent form may need to be signed, either by the patient or a relative. Digitalis should be witheld for 24 - 48 hours prior to the procedure, otherwise serious arrhythmias may occur. As the procedure is essentially a painful one an anaesthetic is usually used. Elective cardioversion is therefore performed on a fasting patient appropriately sedated or anaesthetized. Sedation is usually in the form of 5 - 15 mg of intravenous diazepam (Valium). Of course, if there is VF these points will not need to be considered.

Pads of electrode gel are applied to the right parasternal region and below the angle of the left scapula. Most instruments are capable of recording the ECG through the electrodes used for applying the shock and the rhythm should be monitored and recorded before and after each shock. The precise location of the electrodes ('paddles') is not critical as long as the electrical current traverses the heart. The instrument is charged to the desired energy level. The patient is disconnected from all other electrical appliances including the monitoring ECG and any intravascular pressure measuring device. Since there is a theoretical threat that the electrical current being delivered to the patient could pass through the bed and reach the operator or others, it is a wise practice to have all personnel stand clear of the bed at the moment of discharge. The instrument is discharged by pressing a button on the paddle. It is usually automatically synchronized to deliver the discharge 0.02 s after the peak of the R wave on the ECG. A synchronized discharge of this kind is neither possible or necessary when there is VF.

For the treatment of VF, a shock of 200 joules may be required, although initially a much lower energy shock has merits. The lower the energy of the shock the less the extent of myocardial damage. For other arrhythmias it is best to start with a small shock such as 30 – 50 joules.

Automatic implantable defibrillator

The continuing inability to deal effectively with malignant ventricular arrhythmias outside the hospital setting recently prompted the development of an automatic implantable defibrillator (AID). This device is programmed to monitor the cardiac rhythm continuously, to recognize ventricular tachyarrhythmias, and to deliver corrective defibrillatory discharges when indicated. The main objective of this device is to protect patients at particularly high risk of sudden death from these lethal arrhythmias. Conceptually, it is analogous to an implantable demand pacemaker, except that ventricular arrhythmias instead of asystole are 'sensed', and the delivered pulse has appropriate defibrillatory characteristics. (*Mirowski et al 1980*)

VENOUS CANNULATION

The indication for peripheral intravenous routes falls into three principle routes:

1. To introduce or replace fluids.
2. To administer parenteral medication or nutrition.
3. To monitor central venous pressure (CVP).

Devices available for peripheral venous infusion include a range of metal needles with short lengths of narrow bore plastic tubing ending in latex caps and luer fittings. Cannulae are made in various plastic materials, including Polyvinyl, Polyethylene and Teflon. A dual function device allows for continuous transfusion and/or intermittent injections for drug therapy.

TECHNIQUE

The technique for percutaneous peripheral venous cannulation begins with the choice of a suitable vein. The most convenient site is the dorsum of the hand or in the forearm of the non-dominant side so that the patient's hand can be used normally. Veins at the elbow should be avoided, as the joint would then require immobilization to avoid repeated kinking of the cannula with resulting fracture and leakage. Other possible sites are in the foot, the ankle or the neck.

The procedure should be fully explained to the patient. After clothes have been removed from the limb the vein should be engorged by applying a torniquet or by blood pressure if the arm is allowed to hang downwards. Warming or gentle slapping often promotes dilatation of constricted vessels. The skin should be prepared by shaving excess hair and cleansing with isopropyl alcohol swabs. Careful sterile procedure is important.

Where large cannulae are required in conscious patients, a local anaesthetic may be injected. The skin should be gently stretched so that it can be perforated a short distance away from the vein. In a separate movement, the needle is then passed through the wall of the vein into the lumen. A flashback of blood is often seen at the hub. After a short distance the needle point should be withdrawn into the cannula before it is fully advanced to reduce further risk of perforation. Great care must be taken, as the sharp needle may sever the cannula if it is accidentally withdrawn. The severed part may then embolise to the heart or lung. By placing a finger on the skin, over the end of the cannula, the needle can be completely withdrawn allowing blood to flow back only as far as the hub. If an infusion is required, the line may then be attached. After removing the torniquet, the infusion should be started (turned full on) to confirm that the fluid is infusing correctly. It should then be reduced to the required flow rate.

Cleanliness of the puncture site may be made by a dry non-occlusive dressing. An anti-bacterial spray may be used. The cannula must be fixed securely, as movement may damage it and lead to leakage or inflammation. This can be done with a single piece of broad adhesive plaster. A slit should be made in the plaster to allow ease of access to the side port. Alternatively, three strips of narrow tape can be used. It must be stressed that no plaster or tapes should be attached around the whole circumference of a limb. If an infusion is used, a crêpe bandage may be applied overall and helps to warm the fluid as it flows towards the vein. Splints should be avoided if possible, as movement of the limb discourages stasis of blood and possible thrombosis. The cannula should be flushed with saline and/or heparin to avoid clotting.

Setting up a drip

If a peripheral infusion is required, the sterile infusion fluid and administration sets will also be needed. The label of the fluid container and its contents should be checked beforehand.

The fluid is usually presented in collapsible bags or bottles, but it is sometimes in rigid bottles, which need an air inlet to prevent a vacuum from forming when the fluid flows out into the administration set. To prepare the administration set close the adjustable valve before pushing the connector firmly into the bag or bottle outlet. Squeeze the drip chamber to obtain a fluid level in it (but do not fill). Raise the luer connector (with its sterile cover) above the fluid level and open the valve. The fluid will fill the plastic tubing up to the level in the drip chamber, and by lowering the luer connector to that level the whole tubing will be filled, without the occurrence of any air bubbles. If there are any small bubbles the tube should be held vertical and tapped sharply. This will result in any small bubbles floating to the fluid surfaces. Once the adjustable valve is turned off, the administration set is ready for use.

Conduction disturbances. Atrioventricular block occurs in about 5 – 10% of patients with acute myocardial infarction. First degree AV block is usually of little clinical significance. Second degree AV block (especially Wenckebach type) is potentially dangerous. Pacing is beneficial if the patient does not respond to atropine (for slow ventricular rate). Complete AV block occurs in about 5% of patients. Pacing is usually indicated, and the prognosis is relatively good with inferior infarction, but less so with anterior infarction. All forms of AV block are between two and four times more common with inferior infarction than with anterior. This is because the AV node is supplied by a branch of the right coronary artery, involved in inferior infarction; and is also at times affected by the vagal response, common in inferior infarction. AV block in anterior infarction carries a much higher mortality (about 80%) than in inferior infarction (about 30%).

Asystole. This is usually preceded by conduction disturbances and associated with signs of large infarction together with severe haemodynamic deterioration. It usually responds poorly to therapy.

At this point it is pertinent to discuss the subject of cardiac pacemakers, and their application to treating heart block.

CARDIAC PACEMAKERS

The artificial pacemaker is an electrically operated mechanical device that electronically stimulates the heart muscle to contract. The pace-maker unit consists of an energy source (e.g. batteries) and electrical circuitry, which is connected to an electrode lead terminating against the myocardium. There are both temporary and permanent pacemakers. In temporary pacing the pulse generator is usually located externally in a self-contained battery. In permanent pacing the pulse generator is implanted subcutaneously.

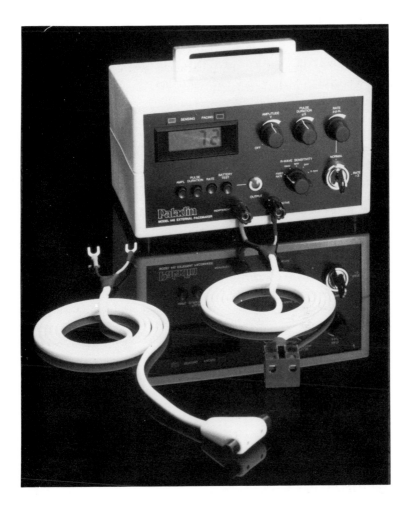

Fig. 59. *External temporary pacemaker.* (Paladin Medical Products Ltd)

On the ECG the pacing stimulus is represented by a sharp spike followed by a complex, similar in appearance to a ventricular ectopic beat.

The two most common modes of pacing are fixed rate and demand (ventricular inhibited). A demand pacemaker is programmed to discharge regular pulses in the absence of spontaneous heart beats or any electrical activity it interprets as heart beats. Fixed rate pacemakers deliver the pulses to the heart at a set rate, irrespective of any activity in the heart.

TEMPORARY (EXTERNAL) PACING

The majority of patients requiring temporary pacing are those in acute illnesses, such as acute myocardial infarction with complete heart block. Other indications include:

Diagnostic uses, as in stress testing.

Prevention and suppression of supraventricular and ventricular tachyarrhythmias which are resistant to drug therapy, by means of overdriving an ectopic focus or by breaking a re-entry circuit with a critically timed impulse.

There are several external pulse generators suitable for temporary pacing. Pacing rate and power output can be adjusted. Facilities for ECG monitoring, fluoroscopy and cardioversion should be readily available.

Routine preparation for surgery is carried out once the patient has given his consent. Following a detailed explanation he will be asked to sign a consent form. The area over the site of insertion of the pacing

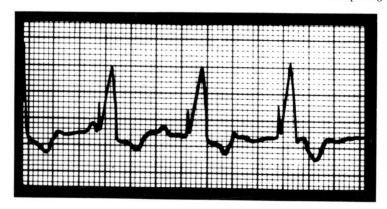

Fig. 60. *'Pacemade' rhythm.*

catheter is shaved. Premedication or a suitable sedative may be given, though the patient is not usually anaesthetized, as his co-operation will be required during the procedure. After the application of a local anaesthetic, the pacing catheter is introduced via a cannula, into the subclavian vein. Alternatively, it may be inserted into the external jugular or antecubital fossa vein. Using fluoroscopy, the catheter is passed into the superior vena cava, the right atrium, the tricuspid valve, and then the right ventricle, where it is lodged against the myocardium. At this stage pacing is instituted and threshold measurements are obtained. The ECG will show the pacing stimulus.

The pacing threshold is the lowest amount of voltage which will reliably produce a ventricular contraction. From the time of positioning the threshold rises for about two weeks and then it plateaus. If the output of the pacemaker is less than the threshold then there will be loss of capture and absence of contraction following each pacing stimulus. The threshold should be measured daily. The output voltage should be around 1.5 V to 2 V above the threshold.

All patients with external pacemakers should be monitored until either a permanent unit is implanted or pacing is discontinued.

PERMANENT (IMPLANTED) PACING

External pacemakers are unsatisfactory for long-term use because of the risk of infection. Permanent pacemakers are indicated in patients with Adams–Stokes syndrome, complete heart block and when syncopal attacks occur. There are several types of implantable pacemakers available. Some use batteries or mercury cells, and are estimated to last five years or more. Batteries or cells can be replaced by making a small surgical incision in the tissue directly over the pacemaker. Lithium implants are now available which are estimated to last eight to ten years.

There are two main ways of implanting a permanent pacing system:

Transvenously into the right ventricle.
Transthoracically and directly fixing the electrode to the outside of the myocardium.

The pacing unit may be implanted in the supramammary region or deep in the sheath of the rectus muscle. Once the complete system is connected together inside the body, the pacemaker starts to function automatically.

The major drawback of this method is that the patient must endure a major operation. However, problems with permanent pacemakers are relatively few.

Periodic ECGs are necessary along with a series of sophisticated tests to determine pacing function, battery power and drainage and mechanical electrode stability. Most pacemakers are designed to slow their rate when there is impending battery exhaustion. A fall of five beats or more per minute indicates the need for replacement.

NURSING CARE

It is important to stress that the nurse remembers to care for the patient and not the machine. Each patient requires individual care and these individualized and specialized needs, which are required for a patient requiring pacing, should be taken into account when care plans are devised.

Preparation

It is important to prepare the patient for his pacemaker. It is useful to give a clear explanation of the reason for it, the actual procedure, and the expected outcome. Even if the doctor has already done this, the patient is likely to have forgotten some of the information. The nurse should include the patient's family in all these discussions, explaining that a pacemaker can help him to return to an active life. She should warn them that although the procedure is successful it is not without complications. If a permanent pacemaker is going to be inserted, the patient could be shown one and allowed to examine it. Some pacemaker manufacturers produce literature especially for these patients, and one should be given to each patient.

Temporary pacing

The basic functions of the nurse caring for this type of patient are to ensure that pacing function is correct, the pacemaker components are safe and that the patient is made comfortable. The patient is initially nursed in bed. The monitor should be observed for any arrhythmias, and these should be dealt with where appropriate. If the pacing wire has been inserted through the antecubital vein, the patient should refrain from excessive movement of the arm. A well-padded arm board helps support and immmobilize the arm. If the pacing wire has been inserted via the subclavian vein it has the advantage of allowing the patient more freedom of movement. Any restrictions imposed upon the patients activities should be explained to him.

The patient who has had a pacemaker inserted usually shows a marked improvement. His mental state improves, blood pressure increases, skin colour improves, and there is often a general feeling of well-being.

The insertion site should be observed in case there is haemorrhage or haematoma; it may be left dry or a light dressing can be applied. The main infections associated with pacing are abscess formation, septicaemia and occasionally bacterial endocarditis. ECG monitoring will indicate whether the pacemaker is functioning properly. A chest X-ray will determine the position of the electrode catheter in the heart. The nurse should check and record the pacing rate, electrical threshold for stimulation and the pacing voltage. On-going patient education should be of prime importance in caring for this type of patient. He should be encouraged to report any symptoms: faintness, chest pain, or hiccups. Analgesia may be required for pain at the insertion site. Sedation should be considered alongside nursing intervention to reduce any patient anxiety. Observations of temperature, pulse and blood pressure are important. The pulse should be compared to the set rate of the pacemaker.

The nurse must familiarize herself with each type of pacemaker, as mechanisms of operation are different in each. All points of contact between each part of the pacemaker should be frequently checked and secured as they are a constant source of malfunction. Most pacemakers can be secured to the bedhead or siderail, and it is important to ensure that a sufficient length of extension lead will allow freedom of movement. Pacemakers should not be placed on bedside lockers or on the floor as they are liable to be dislodged. When a patient is mobilized, a pacemaker of a smaller size can be worn round the neck or abdomen, encased in a pouch.

Complications
The nurse should be aware of complications of pacing which can occur.

Failure to sense the QRS complex can occur, usually due to a poorly positioned pacing electrode, low output voltage, inadequate contact between the electrode and myocardium, or a faulty battery.

Failure to inhibit can occur in demand pacemakers. There is a danger here of the pacing stimulus falling during the recovery or vulnerable phase in the cardiac cycle, sometimes causing ventricular tachycardia or fibrillation.

False inhibiting can also occur in demand pacemakers. The pacemaker waits a longer period than normal before firing. Connections should be closely inspected.

Other points

The immediate environment should be kept as free as possible from electrical hazards. All electronic equipment should be well earthed. If the patient requires defibrillation, the pacemaker must be turned off temporarily.

Following the initial insertion, the rate of the pacemaker is gradually lowered to determine if the patient is pacing on his own. If a demand pacemaker is in place, and there is no artificial pacing for a few days, it can be turned off eventually and removed. However, if the patient is unable to stimulate a satisfactory rate on his own, a permanent pacemaker is usually implanted.

A patient with a permanent pacemaker should be taught to take his own pulse daily, and to notify the doctor of any changes in pulse rate or the occurrence of any symptoms. He may have to limit his activities, if his cardiac output is not sufficient to meet his metabolic needs.

Certain electronic equipment such as microwave ovens interfere with the pacemaker, and the patient should avoid using one. He should be encouraged to comply with any drug regimen, and to attend the out-patient clinic at regular intervals.

Psychological aspects

When a temporary pacemaker is stopped, the patient may become very anxious. He should be reassured that he can return to a normal lifestyle as his heart is fully functioning. Those patients who will require a permanent pacemaker must be prepared in advance. A visit from another patient who already has a permanent pacemaker may be beneficial. A positive approach needs to be adopted by the nurse, and the patient should be encouraged to ask questions about his pacemaker, the effect it will have on his lifestyle, and his family. The latter will also require support from the nurse. Simple explanations and reassurance will often allay any fears the patient may have.

CARDIAC ARREST

Cardiac arrest can be defined as the abrupt cessation of cardiac function due to either ventricular fibrillation or asystole. It may be due to a number of factors, although the commonest cause is acute myocardial infarction. When the heart fails to maintain the cerebral circulation for approximately four minutes, the brain may become irreversibly damaged. Cardiac arrest is not an uncommon emergency in hospital practice, and rapid diagnosis and treatment are essential. The management of cardiac arrest by the nurse (usually, in the CCU) requires rapid decisions (both technical and moral) and speedy actions.

Points to consider

1. Irreversible brain damage often occurs after approximately 4 minutes.

2. The chance of restoring adequate heart rhythm and successfully resuscitating the patient diminishes rapidly with time.

3. 80 - 90% survival can be anticipated on the CCU in patients with primary VF.

4. Survival rates on the ward are approximately 20% lower.

5. Survival rates in the community are virtually nil.

6. External cardiac massage (ECM) can provide only a limited cardiac output.

Waiting for a second opinion, recording the blood pressure, raising the legs and lowering the head have no place in the immediate management of cardiac arrest, as they are a dangerous waste of time.

RECOGNITION OF CARDIAC ARREST

The signs of cardiac arrest are:

1. Abrupt loss of consciousness.
2. Absent carotid and femoral pulses.
3. Absent respirations.

A rapid developing pallor often associated with cyanosis ensues. Pupil dilation is unreliable. Apnoea, gasping, and convulsions may occur later, but are inconsistent signs.

Treatment consists of three phases:

1. External cardiac massage and mouth-to-mouth (cardiopulmonary) resuscitation.

2. Correction of acid-base balance.

3. Assessment and correction of electrolyte imbalance.

External cardiac massage and mouth-to-mouth resuscitation

Since ECM can provide only limited cardiac output, a restoration of adequate heart rhythm should be aimed for. In the absence of evidence to the contrary, it should be assumed that the cardiac arrest is due to VF. An immediate blow to the chest may be attempted as this occasionally restores heart rhythm and takes only seconds. ECM is designed to lead to the ejection of blood from the heart by manual compression of the ventricles between the sternum and the spine, and also to facilitate cyclic passive ventricular filling.

1. The nurse should maintain a clear airway, and ask someone to summon help.

2. The patient should be placed supine on a firm surface.

3. If the blow to the chest fails to elicit any response, cardiac massage should be started, with the heel of one hand on the lower half of the sternum and the other hand applied on top of the first. The arms should be kept straight and the elbows locked. Firm pressure should be applied. The nurse should kneel level with the supine patient to exert maximum pressure. Cardiac massage should consist of one compression per second, therefore allowing adequate time for ventricular filling.

4. Effective ventilation must be carried out; initially by the mouth-to-mouth method. The patient's chin must be retracted and the neck fully extended. The nurse should pinch his nostrils closed with thumb and finger, open his mouth wide, take a deep breath, make an airtight seal over the patient's mouth, and exhale forcefully into his mouth. She should then remove her mouth and allow the patient to exhale passively. She should observe the patient's chest wall for the rise and fall which should occur. If it does not, an obstruction may be present. If so, the patient should be rolled over on his side, his mouth forced open, and an attempt made to remove any foreign body from the back of his throat. Ventilation should be attempted at a rate of 12 per minute.

5. ECM and mouth-to-mouth resuscitation should not be interrupted, as cardiac output increases cumulatively during the first 8 – 10 compressions, and even brief interruptions are detrimental.

It is worth remembering that the brain is more susceptible to ischaemia than anoxia, and therefore ECM should be commenced prior to ventilation if both cannot be instituted simultaneously. In the USA, nurses prefer to initiate ventilation first.

The management of cardiac arrest in the acute setting varies. However, the above steps should be followed until help arrives. In most hospitals, cardiac arrest teams take over resuscitative measures, and apart from those members essential to those measures, other personnel should leave as they only hinder each other.

In the CCU, various equipment is available to the nursing and medical teams. Airways, ambu bags, and endotracheal tubes can be used for assisting ventilation. Oxygen is also readily available. ECG monitoring equipment and a defibrillator are also at hand. If VF is shown to be responsible for the cardiac arrest, DC shock (defibrillation) should be initiated.

Correction of acid-base imbalance

Severe acidosis develops rapidly and should be corrected by giving 100 mmol of sodium bicarbonate intravenously. Subsequent doses are given according to blood gas pH determinations.

Assessment and correction of electrolyte imbalance

Renal failure is not uncommon if cardiac arrest has been prolonged and it is important that the plasma electrolytes are assessed. This applies particularly to plasma potassium. If the plasma potassium level is kept below 4.5 mmol/litre, this may decrease the incidence of VF or other arrhythmias.

CARDIOGENIC SHOCK

This syndrome is considered to be present when hypotension is accompanied by other clinical signs:

1. Hypotension, with systolic blood pressure less than 90 mmHg.
2. Hypoxia and metabolic acidosis.
3. Clinical signs of peripheral 'shutdown': cold and clammy skin and cyanosis of extremities.
4. Oliguria, with urine output less than 20 ml per hour.
5. Dulled sensorium.

About 10 – 15% of patients experiencing infarction develop cardiogenic shock, and the mortality is 90 – 95% irrespective of treatment. Vasopressors (Noradrenaline, Dobutamine, or Dopamine) may be useful as a temporary measure but tend to extend the myocardial damage. Vasodilators (e.g. Nitroprusside) may offer a better result. The use of an intra-aortic balloon pump (IABP) has significantly reduced the mortality, especially when used early in the course of hypotension.

The main objectives of the nurse caring for the patient in shock are astute observation of the patient's general physical and psychological state, recording of physiological parameters, and the prevention of complications. Because of the patient's limited mobility, peripheral vasoconstriction and anoxia, good skin care and position change, and general attention to personal hygiene are important. Because of oliguria, an indwelling urinary catheter may have to be inserted.

INTRA-AORTIC BALLOON PUMP

The use of the IABP has had a major impact on the treatment of cardiogenic shock. The balloon is in the shape of a large catheter which is introduced, via the femoral artery, into the descending aorta. It does not occlude the aorta, but displaces the blood volume by its regular, rapid inflation and deflation. The effect of this pumping action is to raise the diastolic pressure, without raising the systolic pressure, thus increasing coronary blood flow, while reducing oxygen requirement.

The IABP works by means of a process known as counterpulsation, using the ECG as a time reference and main activator. The balloon is inflated during cardiac diastole and deflated when the next period of cardiac systole occurs. Since about 80% of coronary blood flow occurs during diastole, diastolic pressure augmentation produces an increase in coronary blood flow and a diminished degree of left ventricular stroke work. This markedly reduces the workload (up to 40%) because the energy is being injected into the system by the balloon, increasing coronary blood flow (up to 20%).

The indications for using the IABP are:

1. Acute coronary ischaemia (including myocardial infarction).
2. Pre-operative aid for open heart surgery.
3. Cardiogenic shock.

As IABPs are mainly indicated for use in patients with cardiogenic shock, hypotension needs to be considered, since it is a major determinant of the degree of coronary blood flow. Intra-cardiac pressure measurements are ascertained by means of a Swan Ganz catheter. This procedure is performed frequently during the institution of the IABP. To maintain an adequate blood pressure, inotropic agents may need to be used.

The balloon itself is divided into two parts (internal and external) which are connected by a catheter to the pump itself, which is enclosed in a compact, automated machine.

Heart failure

Some degree of heart failure occurs in many patients with myocardial infarction, and does not necessarily require treatment. However, if there is evidence of pulmonary congestion, rapid-acting diuretics such as IV Frusemide are usually effective. Vasodilator drugs may be advocated. Drugs such as sodium nitroprusside (Nipride) reduce cardiac work and improve left ventricular performance, with an increase in cardiac output.

Papillary muscle rupture and dysfunction

This is usually the underlying cause of mitral incompetence, which occurs in 10 – 20% of patients with infarction. In a small proportion of patients a papillary muscle rupture results in severe heart failure. Surgery will need to be considered.

Cardiac rupture

This is most likely to occur during the first week after the onset of symptoms. It may be present clinically with a sudden disappearance of the pulse, blood pressure and consciousness, while the ECG continues to show sinus rhythm; this combination of death with a continuing ECG is almost diagnostic.

Pericarditis

Acute pericarditis develops in about 20% of patients, usually on the second to third day. Pain is the dominant feature, and is often mistaken for a recurrence of infarction. Usually, the only treatment required is analgesia. Indomethacin is a very effective drug in treating pericarditis.

Ventricular aneurysms

These occur in 10 – 20% of patients. The term *ventricular asynergy* describes disorders of ventricular function. Two forms of this are *dyskinesis* (local paradoxical wall movement) and *akinesis* (local absence of wall movement). Ventricular function is impaired by these disorders because normally functioning myocardial fibres must shorten. ECG findings include maintained ST segment elevations after the acute stage. Ventricular aneurysms may be responsible for persistent ventricular arrhythmias such as VT.

Embolism

The extent to which pulmonary embolism occur in infarct patients is not certain because of their rapid mobilization. However, the possibility of it occurring should be considered whenever a patient with infarction develops right heart failure.

Systemic embolism is particularly liable to occur in those patients with atrial fibrillation.

Shoulder–hand syndrome

A few patients have pain and limitation of movement of the left arm and shoulder following infarction. It is probably related to the immobility imposed during the early phase of the acute illness.

POST-CARDIAC-INJURY SYNDROME

It has recently been recognized that a number of disorders which are identical in their clinical manifestations, may appear under a variety of circumstances. They have one common feature: previous myocardial injury. The syndrome may follow a cardiac operation (post-pericardiotomy syndrome), myocardial infarction (Dressler's syndrome), or following trauma of the heart.

CLINICAL FEATURES

Pain

This is the principal symptom which usually develops after an interval of 2 – 4 weeks following the cardiac injury. The outstanding features are:

Pericarditis
Pleuritis
Pneumonitis
Fever

The illness usually subsides within a month. Apart from adequate analgesia, usually no other treatment is necessary. If the illness is severe, steroid therapy is usually beneficial.

REHABILITATION

INTRODUCTION

The purpose of rehabilitation is to minimize the impact of the infarct on the patients lifestyle and psyche. The nurse should prepare the patient for rehabilitation from the start. A brief chat and giving out a booklet is no substitute for nurse-patient discussion. Many patients are badly informed and do not have a clear idea of what has happened to them, and what can be expected of them in the future. Patients often feel that they 'were kept in the dark', 'unaware they had had a coronary', 'unable to rest enough', 'anxious', and 'not satisfied with care'. Therefore, the first detailed discussion should take place soon after the infarct, as soon as the patient is free from pain and the acute phase is over. The nurse should sit down and explain frankly to the patient what has happened and what is expected of him in the future. She should take a realistic and optimistic approach (most mortalities occur before hospital admission) during discussion with the patient concerning his progressive increase in activity. Early ambulation and discharge are encouraged as these reduce depression as well as physical weakness and loss of muscle tone. In certain hospitals patients are allowed to sit out of bed on the day of admission provided they are free of pain and significant arrhythmias.

The nurse plays the most important role in the rehabilitation of the patient and should participate more in the planning of these programmes. Little attention has been given to the home care of the patient. In the UK, district nursing services (in conjunction with CCU staff) should make provision to make regular visits into the patient's home.

Rehabilitation of the coronary patient is accepted by most nurses (and doctors) as part of their responsibilities. Few doubt that there is the need for some form of organized and supervized rehabilitation to restore the patient to an optimum level of recovery. Yet despite this agreement, rehabilitation of the coronary patient is not achieved throughout the country.

It is important that a positive, optimistic approach is adopted by the nurse during the rehabilitation of coronary patients. Rehabilitation should begin on admission of the patient to the coronary care unit, with explanation and discussion, both for the patient and for his family. From early convalescence in hospital, the patient and spouse should be encouraged that a return to normal physical activity within a matter of a few weeks is not only possible, but also safe and beneficial. Bad advice such as 'don't overdo things' or 'take things easy' is responsible for the delayed return to work and to a normal lifestyle.

REHABILITATION ON THE WARD

It has already been stated that when the patient is transferred from the CCU to the ward anxiety levels are increased. It is vital that the nurse appreciates this and provides support during this transition. Unfortunately, ward nurses tend to perceive these patients as less acutely ill than they actually are. The nurse therefore needs to thoroughly and accurately assess the patient and intervene with any appropriate nursing action. Nursing care plans should be aimed at achieving full and rapid mobilization and a return home. The patient should be able to reach the activity level required for self-care by the time he returns home.

When the nurse plans her care for the patient she should take into account that he is often the best judge of how much activity he should do. The major objectives of nursing care are to assist the patient and his family to:

1. Understand, accept, and adapt to his illness (and any limitations).
2. Take part in his recovery and rehabilitation.
3. Provide him with support and guidance.

A large proportion of patients are not rehabilitated because of psychological rather than physiological reasons. An increase in anxiety and depression is frequently noticeable when the patient is confronted by the uncertainties and minor physical symptoms that accompany mobilization and the return home. Depression and anxiety, irritability, fatigue, and poor concentration are expected in the months after infarction. However, some of these behavioural changes can be minimized or averted by a satisfactory hospital rehabilitation programme. For example group therapy sessions and relaxation classes are ideal methods of assisting rehabilitation.

Within a flexible and positive framework a plan can be drawn up for each patient's rehabilitation.

A detailed discussion of this topic can be found elsewhere (*Wilson-Barnett 1979*).

MOBILIZATION AND DISCHARGE ADVICE

Progress in early rehabilitation has been greatly assisted by the use of the metabolic equivalent (Met.). One Met. is defined as the energy expenditure per kilogram per minute of the average 70 kg individual sitting quietly in a chair. This amounts to about 1.4 cal. per min. or 3.5 – 4 ml of oxygen per min. The table below provides a list of activities which have been assigned measurements in Mets. It is of interest to note that using a bed-pan requires one third again as much energy as using a bedside commode. Average middle-aged men, three months or more after an uncomplicated infarct, are capable of performing at a level of 8 – 9 Mets. This includes running at 5.5 mph, cycling at 13 mph, and 'non-competitive' squash. If less than ordinary activity produces symptoms in the post-infarct patient, then his capacity is about 4 Mets.

TABLE 2: Energy expenditure for self-care activities for a 70 kg male

Activity	Mets
Sitting	1
Eating	1
Dressing/undressing	2
Washing hands and face	2
Bedside commode	3
Walking 2.5 mph	3
Using bed-pan	4
Walking downstairs	4.5
Walking 3.5 mph	5.5

TABLE 3: Energy expenditure for daily activities for a 70 kg male

Activity	Mets
Mowing lawn by hand	6.5
Shovelling	7
Driving car	2
Squash	8.5
Swimming 18 m/min	4
Gardening	4.5
Ironing while standing	3.5
Sexual intercourse	5 – 6

THE TEACHING CARE PLAN

Although patient teaching is an important nursing function, there is much evidence which shows that effective and consistent teaching is not being accomplished by nurses. Yet, patients are becoming much more knowledgeable in health matters and are demanding more information about their illness, treatment, and future events.

In order that the teaching–learning process can function effectively, the patients' readiness and motivation to learn needs to be determined. Patients' attitudes may affect learning, as they are difficult to change; knowledge of facts does not necessarily change attitudes or behaviour.

Teaching patients

The nurse is in an ideal position to teach patients. She knows the patient's diagnosis, treatment, and prognosis; she is with the patient 24 hours a day; and she is often better able to communicate with the patient and see things from his point of view.

Patients often want information about things that are done to them and why; what to expect after treatment; more information about nursing procedures; and more discharge and rehabilitation information. They usually require simple answers to their questions and fewer medical terms. Many patients do not ask questions because they do not know what to ask, how to ask, when to ask, or whom to ask. If patient teaching is to be beneficial the patient needs to perceive the nurse as a teacher. Teaching is better if it is structured rather than unstructured, when it is repeated more than once, and when it is written as well as verbal. Group teaching is also an effective and more efficient method than individual teaching. However, for this to work properly, the members of the group need to be carefully selected so that they have similar learning needs. It is pointless to include coronary patients with postoperative coronary artery bypass graft patients. (*Pohl, 1965*)

The use of audio-visual aids are becoming increasingly important in patient teaching. Pamphlets on coronary's, high-blood pressure, etc. are a valuable teaching aid.

Teaching patients' families

An integral part of the patient's care and rehabilitation is the education of his family so that they play a helpful rather than a detrimental role. The family can have a direct influence on the patient by accepting and understanding his condition, adapting to it, and modifying his lifestyle. They should be involved in most, if not all, patient teaching so that they have the necessary information about heart disease and the patient's medication. It may be true that patient and family teaching cannot be accomplished adequately during the hospital stay. More information can be learned and retained and more problems can be identified and resolved after the patient has been discharged from the hospital.

Teaching content

Factors that need to be considered when deciding upon the teaching content are the patient's level of knowledge and education, and social and cultural factors. Major factors which interfere with learning are increased anxiety, denial and depression. (*Cohen 1981*)

The content of the teaching care plan for the coronary patient needs to include:

1. Information on a heart attack
2. Activity (general, sexual, and work)
3. Diet
4. Medications
5. Risk factors

Other areas specific to individual patients such as pacemakers, diabetes, etc. should also be covered.

Patient information

Many patients feel that they are not being told what they want to know. This is usually due to:

Lack of time

Nurses' attitude. Some nurses still think that it is wrong for patients to know too much about their illness. To them, 'good patients' are those who do what they are told without question; while those who demand information are 'troublesome patients'. Most patients nowadays want more information than they are usually given. The apparent reluctance of nurses to supply this probably partly derives from their unconscious need to dominate patients.

Patients' submissiveness and forgetfulness

Improving patient information

The nurse should realize that she is frequently the person expected to satisfy the patient's need for information about his illness. She needs to give information in a friendly way and encourage the patient to be an equal partner in aiming for his eventual recovery. She should introduce herself, sit down, and chat to the patient in an unhurried manner.

Better verbal information. Patients more easily remember things said in simple language, and earlier statements better than later ones. Repetition also increases recall, as does specific rather than general advice. However, whatever is said by the nurse is often forgotten by the patient.

Written information. Supplementing verbal with written information increases patient compliance. Simple, printed pamphlets are a great asset.

Encouragement of patients' question. Nurses should actively encourage patients to ask any questions.

Information on a heart attack

The first area to be considered in explaining to the patient about his coronary is a brief simple description. Pamphlets and drawings are often very useful. The British Heart Foundation produces much literature in this area, and they have an excellent series of layman's guides: 'Heart Research Series' (No. II: 'The heart and its problems', is ideal).

Information should include the size of the problem of IHD, about atheroma, terminology, risk factors, and an explanation of the common investigations — ECG and blood tests.

ACTIVITIES

Introduction

Habitual physical activity has been associated with a decreased occurrence of IHD in several population studies, but it has not been shown whether exercise alters the occurrence or progress of the disease. Dynamic exercises, however, can be recommended as a rehabilitative measure after infarction. It may:

1. Improve physical work capacity and cardiac performance.
2. Improve mood and morale.
3. Facilitate an early return to work.

GENERAL ACTIVITIES

Patients should be encouraged to gradually increase their activity levels, but not excessively. However, as already stated they are usually the best judges of how much they can do. They should be prepared for any 'weak feelings' which may accompany increases in activity.

Before going home the patient will have been able to walk upstairs. After a few weeks at home the patient should be able to do light household and gardening chores, and should be physically active prior to returning to work. It is important to encourage patients to exercise daily, and to stress that a lack of exercise is harmful rather than beneficial. The best form of exercise during convalescence is walking. The patient should be encouraged to walk for about 10 minutes a day, which should be increased until the patient is walking for one to one and a half hours a day. Golf, swimming, cycling, etc. should be encouraged once the patient feels well enough. It is usually wise not to drive a car for the first month after leaving hospital, as this can be quite stressful. A history of infarction is a contraindication to holding a HGV licence. A PSV licence is also usually withdrawn.

The patient is safe to travel by air as soon as the period of convalescence is over. However, long flights are inadvisable initially. Airline medical staff are very willing to give advice and help to patients with any of these problems.

If the patient encounters any difficulties at home he should be encouraged to visit his GP as soon as possible.

SEXUAL ACTIVITY

Sexual counselling should be an integral part of the cardiac rehabilitation programme. Therefore, the nurse requires a knowledge of both human sexuality and IHD. The energy expenditure during coitus for long-married couples is equivalent to that of climbing stairs, therefore the risk of infarction is low. In fact, depression through a lack of positive encouragement to resume sexual activity is far more dangerous than the actual activity. However, a combination of illicit affairs, emotional outbursts, alcohol and heavy meals may precipitate reinfarction or even death. Stressful sexual situations are more likely to cause trouble than domestic ones. A sexual activity programme is workable only if each partner gives and receives pleasure. Because of the long-term mutual commitment of marriage, sexual activity is of great importance, forming a strong link in the inter-relationship between all the components of marriage. Ordinary marital intercourse can and should be restarted as soon as moderate exercise is restarted. (*Thompson 1980b*)

Teaching and counselling

The nurse should be aware that many people have conflicts about sex, and are unwilling to talk directly about this. Through counselling their anxiety can be reduced.

It is important to include both partners in a non-threatening environment where the couple can speak freely. They should be informed of the effects of the illness on sexual functioning. The primary objectives here are to restore the couple to pre-illness functioning, educate them about human sexuality, and facilitate their communication. Education about sexuality should take into account the intellectual and developmental level of the couple.

With counselling, it has been found that patients revelaed fear of another infarction during coitus, body image changes, anxiety on the part of the spouse, and the belief that the initial loss of sexual interest and erectile difficulties were permanent. Nurses as educators and counsellors are in a prime position to alter false opinions and give corrective information. Certainly patients have a right to know what is happening to them and how they can help themselves.

Nurses who feel uneasy, embarrassed or uncomfortable in discussing sex with patients may benefit from attending workshops and study days. A true rapport with the patient is essential to a trusting, honest and giving relationship. The subject of sex should never be ignored by the nurses and doctors.

Research results have shown that coitus culminating in orgasm may produce transient tachycardia, hypertension and hyperventilation. Pressures in the region of 230/130 mmHg have been recorded at orgasm in normotensive individuals, but both the heart rate and blood pressure fall rapidly to pre-coital levels after orgasm. The effects of coitus on the heart should be explained to the patient and spouse. There seems to be little difference in heart load between various coital positions, or between coitus and masturbation. Abstinence from coitus is probably advisable for one month after infarction, but ordinary marital intercourse should be restarted as soon as moderate exercise is restarted. The period will depend on the patient's progress which may be quantitatively assessed by exercise testing. If the patient complains of angina or breathlessness during coitus, a Holter monitor will distinguish between anxiety and decompensation. A prophylactic coronary dilator (GTN) will usually suppress true angina.

RETURN TO WORK

The return to work usually gives the patient increased self-satisfaction, restored self-respect, and relief from financial worries. However, many employers believe that these patients cannot or should not work at all. Compensation and Social Security payments create a disincentive to return to work, as does doctors advice 'to lay off work and take things easy for a few months'. Several factors have been identified which affect a patient's return to work. Initially, the severity of myocardial damage will affect work return success. The more medical complications from the infarction resulting in heart damage will provide less probability of a return to work, as will advanced working age, a stressful work situation, sporadic work record, family instability, and lack of knowledge about heart disease.

A multidisciplinary approach is often needed with work problems, which includes the nurse, doctor, social workers, disablement resettlement officer, and employer. Initially the patient may be advised to return to work on a part-time basis, and occasionally to lighter work. A few patients involved in heavy manual work may need to change their occupation, though this is not always acceptable to the patient, especially in the present industrial and economic climate.

DIET

It must be appreciated that it has not been proven that dietary modification can prevent ischaemic heart disease. Hyperlipidaemia is certainly associated with IHD and may even be one of the causes, but the genesis of this in more than 95% of the general population is simply not understood. Regarding a reduction of cholesterol, drugs and diet have been ineffective in either limitation or prevention of IHD. In fact, some authorities believe that a low-fat diet may not lead to a reduced risk of IHD, but may actually increase the risk.

The prevention of obesity, however, is a different matter. This is the single most important dietary measure likely to improve the individual's health.

The nurse should possess the knowledge and skills necessary to meet the nutritional requirements of the patient. It is clearly important that advice given by the nurse be both as accurate and consistent as possible. In view of the lack of evidence it is wrong for nurses to counsel patients on how to follow a low-saturated-fat, low-cholesterol, increased-polyunsaturated diet if the patient has never been used to such a regimen. Other factors are more important than a fat diet. Nurses as educators and counsellors should be aware of the fats controversy.

One of the major problems is not in the giving of advice to patients and their relatives, but in achieving appropriate behavioural responses which are in their own best interests.

MEDICATIONS

Medications and drug compliance are considered separately at the end of the book (pp. 254–255). However, the patient should be taught by the nurse to be able to identify his medication, understand the basic action of it, and know the number of tablets to take and when to take them. Patient teaching should also extend to the family as this may improve patient compliance.

One ideal way of teaching the patient about his medication involves the use of a small file or index card with the patient's tablet(s) affixed. The medication's name, dose, time to be taken, action, and side effects are written on the card. This should then be given to the patient to be stored with his medications at home, thus serving as a reminder, and also providing important information.

RISK FACTORS

Teaching the patient about risk factors presumes that the person will give up 'bad habits' on being informed about the relative risks involved for IHD. However, health education (individualized or by mass media) is not sufficient by itself to produce desired changes in health behaviour. Many centres now use behavioural approaches in dealing with risk reduction. These behavioural approaches generally refer to behaviour modification techniques. Because these techniques are too complex to be considered here, the reader is advised to refer to standard psychology texts dealing with behaviour therapy.

CORONARY-PRONE BEHAVIOUR PATTERN

The coronary-prone behaviour pattern is best assessed by observing the patient in action. Type A behaviour is seen in those individuals who are chronically impatient, who are always mentally active, who can converse only on topics that interest him, who is competitive, and who feels guilty for relaxing. The type B person is more relaxed and unhurried, yet may accomplish as much work in a given time as the type A. The type A patient will want to return to his usual lifestyle as soon as possible. He will probably want work bringing into hospital, and may make sexual overtones towards female nursing staff. He is often excessively demanding and quite disruptive in the ward situation. The nurse can often divert some of this patient's energy towards therapeutic goals, by making him a partner and friend in his recovery process. The patient must be made to realize that his behaviour is part of his health problem. Once this is understood and accepted, it may be possible to help the patient change his behaviour.

DISCHARGE HOME

The transition from hospital to home is a traumatic one for the patient and his family. It is a time when the nurse should ensure continuity of care and family and patient support. Unfortunately, this ideal situation hardly exists at all. The role of the nurse as a leading member of the primary health care team is a unique one which could, and should, play a much more active part. The district nurse could continue patient education and assist the patient and family in coping with the increased level of anxiety and other manifestations which usually occur during the first week at home. Obviously, communication between the coronary care nurse and the district nurse needs to be consistent, accurate, free and open-ended.

The district nurse can play an important role in teaching, counselling and evaluation of nursing care plans, which are all necessary if continuity of care is to be consistent.

A multi-disciplinary health team approach is advantageous as it combines skills of professionals and provides continuity between hospital and community care. Management in a clinic rather than by a GP, has been found to halve the incidence of non-fatal re-infarction and all new coronary events (*Vedin et al 1976*)

USEFUL INFORMATION FOR THE PATIENT

Many patients often request further information concerning their coronary. Nurses should encourage them to read such material as much of the information given in hospital is often already forgotten. They should be advised to choose factual, up-to-date literature which is easy to understand. Such literature includes:

TABLE 4:

Patient teaching programme items. Problem: Myocardial infarction

	Date	Initial	Need for further teaching		Comment
			Yes	No	
1. *Adjustment to CCU:*					
(a) Purpose of CCU					
(b) Explanation of monitor					
(c) I.V. infusion & Drugs					
(d) Oxygen					
(e) ECG; venepuncture; X-Rays					
(f) Diet					
(g) Activity					
(h) Visiting arrangements					
2. *Adjustment to transfer from CCU:*					
(a) Constant observation no longer necessary					
(b) Activities as prescribed					
(c) Plan for teaching programme					
3. *Information needed for adaptation to disease:*					
(a) Basic anatomy & function of heart					
(b) Development of IHD					
(c) Myocardial infarction including: Risk factors Warning signs of coronary Healing process in relation to physical activity					

Checklist

Patient teaching programme items. Problem: Myocardial infarction

	Date	Initial	Need for further teaching		Comments
			Yes	No	
(d) Psychological response to coronary: Individual or group discussion Individual discussion with patient and family					
4. *Plans for follow-up care* *Information re:* (a) Discharge medication (b) Activity: general, sexual, and work (c) Diet (d) Symptoms to be reported (e) Rehabilitation exercises (f) Clinic or GP appointments (g) Community follow-up help resources					
5. *Special areas for teaching:* e.g. Pacemakers					
6. *Educational materials:* e.g. basic pamphlets					

For each item listed, the date of teaching and the nurse's name are recorded, as is the need for further patient education on that topic and the nurse's comments regarding the patient's comprehension.

1. British Heart Foundation. *Heart Research Series pamphlets* (1980). Published in a series of eleven, they are written for patients and their families, and cover every aspect of ischaemic heart disease. They are obtainable from the BHF, 57 Gloucester Place, London. W1H4DH.

2. J.P. Shillingford, *Coronary Heart Disease: The Facts.* (1980) Oxford. Written by a distinguished cardiologist, this book should be recommended to all patients.

3. B. Phibbs, *The Human Heart: A Guide to Heart Disease.* (1975) Mosby. Written by five American physicians and a nurse, this book is intended to give patients more knowledge about the heart and its diseases. Although primarily intended for the USA, it will benefit many patients and nurses in the UK. It is well illustrated.

PROGNOSIS

About 60% of deaths from acute myocardial infarction occur during the first few hours, with an additional 10% mortality within the next two days. Although the impact of coronary care units has reduced in-hospital mortality by about a third, it only reduces overall mortality by a few percent.

Once in hospital, the patient's progress is strongly related to age. Mortality is about 10% in 50 year olds increasing to over 50% after the age of 70. The prognosis is better in those patients who do not have hypertension, angina, or heart failure.

Overall, 80 – 90% of patients survive at least one year, and 60% survive ten years.

SUDDEN DEATH

Sudden death resulting from IHD has only recently begun to receive attention. Approximately 40% of all patients sustaining acute myocardial infarction die, and most of these suddenly. The greatest incidence of mortality is within fifteen minutes of the attack. 50% of all deaths take place within two hours of the onset of symptoms (40% during the first hour and 10% during the second hour). Comparatively few die if they survive the twelve hours following the attack.

The exact cause of death in those who die suddenly is uncertain, as most of the deaths are unwitnessed. It is apparent that over half of the subjects who die suddenly had a previous history of myocardial infarction or angina. These subjects may complain of sudden chest pain or breathlessness at the time, or the victim may die so suddenly that he is seen to collapse and die without having complained of any symptoms. Many die in their sleep. The majority of deaths are due to ventricular fibrillation (VF), often without any preceding ventricular arrhythmia, heart failure or cardiogenic shock. Myocardial ischaemia is probably the most common cause of VF. If intensive care was applied early enough it is apparent that a substantial proportion of all deaths could be prevented.

PREVENTION OF SUDDEN DEATH

The vast majority of these attacks will prove fatal because of the unavailability of the necessary equipment and trained personnel. Therefore, prevention of sudden death seems obvious (Julian and Campbell 1981). Prevention depends on at least two developments:

1. The identification of those at high risk from ventricular arrhythmias, and the availability of therapeutic measures to prevent VF.
2. The understanding of mechanisms and pathophysiological factors that are involved in causing VF.

An example of high risk patients are those who have recovered from a recent myocardial infarction, as the mortality remains increased for about six months thereafter. Continuous oral anti-arrhythmic therapy has been advocated for all those at risk of sudden death.

ANTI-ARRHYTHMIC THERAPY

Numerous studies have been and are being conducted to discover whether the incidence of sudden death can be reduced. Several drugs have been investigated, including clofibrate, the beta-blockers, sulphinpyrazone and aspirin. There is so far no unequivocal evidence that the routine use of any of these drugs is beneficial. The ideal anti-arrhythmic agent would be one that is effective against a wide variety of important tachyarrhythmias, requires only infrequent administration, and is largely free of notable side effects.

Apart from drugs, other efforts are being made to reduce the incidence of sudden death, including surgical methods. An implantable automatic defibrillator has been described that the patient may use to correct his own ventricular arrhythmia.

REFERENCES

Abdellah, F.G. (1972) *The nursing role in the coronary care system.* In: *Textbook of Coronary Care* (Ed: L.E. Meltzer and A.J. Dunning). Amsterdam: Excerpta med.

Adgey, A.A.J. (1980) Coronary patient — early treatment. *Br. Heart J.* *44*, 357.

Ashworth, P. (1980) *Care to communicate.* London: RCN.

Bergman, G. Daly, K., Atkinson, L., Rothman, M., Richardson, P.J., Jackson, G. & Jewitt, D.E. (1981) Prostacyclin: haemodynamic and metabolic effects in patients with coronary artery disease. *Lancet, i,* 569.

Burch, P.R.J. (1980) Review: ischaemic heart disease: epidemiology, risk factors and cause. *Cardiovasc. Res., 14,* 307.

Cassem, N.H. & Hackett, T.P. (1975) Stress on the nurse and therapist in the ICU and CCU. *Heart and Lung, 4,* 252.

Cattell, M. & Balcon, R. (1981) *Coronary artery surgery.* In: *Recent Advances in Cardiology* (Ed: J. Hamer & D.J. Rowlands). Edinburgh: Churchill Livingstone.

Cohen, S.A. (1981) Patient education: a review of the literature. *J. adv. Nurs., 6,* 11.

Joint Working Party of the Royal College of Physicians of London and the British Cardiac Society (1976) Prevention of coronary heart disease. *J. R. Col. Phys., 10,* 213.

Julian, D.G. & Campbell, R.W.F. (1981) *Sudden coronary death.* In: *Recent advances in Cardiology* (Ed. J. Hamer & D.J. Rowlands). Edinburgh: Churchill Livingstone.

Kannel, W.B., Dawber, T.R., Friedman, G.D., Glennon, W.E. & McNamara, P.M. (1964) Risk factors in coronary heart disease (Framingham Study). *Ann. intern. Med., 61,* 888.

Marriott, H.J.L. & Fogg, G. (1970) Constant monitoring for cardiac dysrhythmias and blocks. *Mod. Concepts cardiovasc. Dis., 39,* 103.

Maseri, A. (1981) The revival of coronary spasm. *Am. J. Med., 70,* 752.

Mather, H.G., Pearson, N.G., Read, K.L.Q., Shaw, D.B., Steed, G.R., Thorne, M.G., Jones, S., Guerrier, C.J., Eraut, C.D., McHugh, P.M., Chowdhury, N.R., Jafary, M.H. & Wallace, T.J. (1971) Acute myocardial infarction: home and hospital treatment. *Br. med. J., 3,* 334.

McMichael, J. (1979) Fats and atheroma: an inquest. *Br. med. J., 1,* 173.

Mirowski, M., Mower, M.M. & Reid, P.R. (1980) The automatic implantable defibrillator. *Am. Heart J., 100,* 1089.

Pohl, M.L. (1965) Teaching activities of the nursing practitioner. *Nurs. Res.*, *14*, 4.

Thompson, D.R. (1980) Fats and heart disease: a point for controversy. *Nurs. Times*, *76*, 1360.

Thompson, D.R. (1980) Sexual activity following acute myocardial infarction in the male. *Nurs. Times*, *76*, 1965.

U.S. Senate Committee on Nutrition and Human Needs (1977) *Dietary goals for the United States.*

Wilson-Barnett, J. (1979) A review of research into the experience of patients suffering from coronary thrombosis. *Int. J. nurs. Stud.*, *16*, 183.

World Health Organization Working Group on the Development of Coronary Care in the Community (1979). *Review of developments in coronary care in the last 5 years.* Regional Office for Europe, Brussels. ICP/CVD 003(9)

Yudkin, J. (1972) Sucrose and cardiovascular disease. *Proc. Nutr. Soc.*, *31*, 331.

8
Hypertension

Hypertension is very difficult to define. The definition depends upon the arbitrary limits we put on normality. For example, a patient with the common arbitrary upper limit of 140/90 mmHg classified as hypertensive on one occasion might be normal on the next or vice versa. For this reason a person should have recordings of their blood pressure obtained on at least three separate intervals over a period of weeks.

The World Health Organization (WHO) has defined 'hypertension' as blood pressure of 160/95 mmHg or above. However blood pressure (BP) readings of 140/90 or above are considered elevated by most clinicians, for individuals under the age of 50 years. For persons older than 50 years of age, BP readings of 160/95 mmHg or higher are considered elevated by most clinicians.

It is interesting to note that blood pressure tends to be lower when recorded by nurses than when recorded by a doctor. (*Richardson and Robinson 1971*)

The prevalence of hypertension varies with different populations and different geographical locations. The best long-term epidemiological data to date is that of the 'Framingham Study' in the U.S.A., where random sample of 5000 subjects was followed for about 20 years. It was found that about one half of the population dying from cardiovascular disease had previously been hypertensive. Environment and occupation have important effects on hypertension. (*Kannel and Dawber 1974*)

TYPES OF HYPERTENSION

It is clear that arterial hypertension does not have a single cause. Such cases are then referred to as *essential* (*primary* or *idiopathic*) *hypertension*. This accounts for 95% of cases. In a few cases (5%), the cause may be defined, such as an endocrine or renal abnormality, then known as *secondary hypertension*.

In all cases of hypertension a small proportion are recognized where the level of pressure suddenly rises. The disease is then said to have passed from a slowly progressive form, misnamed 'benign', to an accelerated form named malignant, since the majority of patients will die within six to twelve months, if untreated. Clinically the hallmarks of malignant hypertension are papilloedema and proteinura.

CLASSIFICATION BY AETIOLOGY

Essential hypertension

This is defined as high blood pressure without evident organic cause.

Secondary hypertension

This is defined as hypertension with identifiable cause. The main causes are:

1. Renal disease: renal artery stenosis, polycystic disease, pyelonephritis, renal embolism, analgesic nephropathy, renal transplantation.
2. Endocrine disease: Cushing's syndrome (adrenal cortical tumour or hyperplasia), aldosteronism (Conn's syndrome), Phaeochromocytoma.
3. Coarctation of the aorta.
4. Toxaemia of pregnancy.
5. Oral contraception.
6. Intracerebral lesions.
7. Acute porphyria.

CONTROL OF BLOOD PRESSURE

Blood pressure is normally regulated by two mechanisms; neurogenic and humoral.

Neurogenic mechanism

Vasoconstriction is mediated by the beta-adrenergic nerves (of the sympathetic system). The control centre is the vasomotor centre in the medulla oblongata. A normal level of blood pressure is maintained by reflex arcs derived from *stretch receptors*, which are special pressure-sensitive nerve endings located in the aortic arch and *carotic sinus.*

Humoral mechanism

An enzyme *renin*, is produced in the kidney by cells near the point where the blood vessels enter the glomerulus, the *juxta-glomerular apparatus*. The main stimulus for renin release appears to be a reduced renal perfusion pressure. Renin converts the plasma protein *angiotensinogen* to a physiologically inactive *Angiotensin I*, and this is further changed in the lung to active *Angiotensin II*. This substance is the most potent vasoconstrictor known. It also stimulates the adrenal cortex to release *aldosterone.* Aldosterone causes sodium and water retention, increasing the plasma volume and therefore raising the blood pressure.

The increased output of aldosterone reduces the production of renin so that there is a negative feed-back mechanism, which tends to maintain a steady effective blood volume and blood pressure.

Pathology

Medial hypertrophy of the arterioles with thickening of the intima is widespread, involving the kidneys, brain and other organs. Hypertrophy of the left ventricle is followed by dilatation, and as the blood pressure rises in the left atrium and pulmonary veins there is consequent pulmonary hypertension and hypertrophy of the right heart.

Hypertension appears to accelerate the development of atheromatous lesions of the arteries. These lesions and intimal thickening result in ischaemia of the kidneys which then show coarse scarring. The kidneys may be considerably shrunken.

Clinical features

Hypertension is frequently discovered on routine examination of apparently healthy subjects. The danger of hypertension is that it is a disease which exists almost without symptoms until some catastrophe occurs, when it may present with serious complications such as stroke, heart failure, or myocardial infarction.

Dyspnoea. This appears to be the only specific symptom, probably due to left ventricular failure.

Some patients may complain of dizziness, blurred vision and poor mental concentration.

Pulses. Pulsus alternans and paroxysmal atrial fibrillation may occur.

Auscultation. A pre-systolic heart sound may be heard.

Haemorrhages and exudates (which look like cotton wool patches) may be seen in the fundus of the eye by using an ophthalmoscope.

Sustained untreated hypertension results in arterial damage. Cerebral haemorrhage and thrombosis, retinal haemorrhage and blindness, renal arterial damage with progressive failure, and ischaemic heart disease are all consequences of raised arterial pressure.

Risk factors
Sex. Women seem to withstand hypertension better than men.

Lipids. Raised plasma lipids are considered by many to be a risk factor.

Other factors. Cigarette smoking, ECG evidence of left ventricular hypertrophy, and glucose intolerance are important adverse factors.

Investigations
Unlike most common conditions there is little agreement about the extent to which hypertension should be investigated. It is important that the diagnosis of hypertension is based on adequate clinical assessment.

Blood pressure. Careful recording and accurate charting of the blood pressure is very important.

Pulses. The femoral pulses should be palpated for the characteristic poor volume and delayed impulse of coarctation of the aorta.

ECG. This may show evidence of ventricular hypertrophy.

Chest X-Ray. This may show evidence of heart failure.

Urinalysis. Routine urinalysis for albumin, cells and culture may show evidence of a renal cause.

Blood urea, creatinine, and electrolytes. An increased sodium and depleted potassium level associated with considerable potassium excretion in the urine suggests the presence of an adenoma of the adrenal glands (Conn's syndrome).

Vanillylmandelic acid (VMA). A simple screening test for the presence of VMA — an end-product of adrenaline and noradrenaline metabolism — in the urine is useful for diagnosing phaeochromocytoma.

Intravenous pyelography (IVP). Intravenous pyelography, renal arteriography, renal biopsy, and isotope scans should be reserved only if there is a clinical hint of renal disease.

TREATMENT

This is undoubtedly indicated if there is malignant hypertension. If the hypertension is secondary, the primary cause must be dealt with, but in the majority of cases treatment is directed to control of the blood pressure itself and its effects.

It has been demonstrated that the prognosis of hypertension is greatly improved if the blood pressure can be maintained below 150/90 mmHg. All patients whose blood pressure persistently exceeds this level require drug treatment.

Before initiating drug treatment, surgically correctable disorders such as coarctation of the aorta, renal artery stenosis, and phaeochromocytoma, should be excluded.

Drug treatment requires careful consideration. Compliance with treatment is a real problem, once-a-day regimens being more closely followed by the patient than those involving a number of drugs at several different times of day.

About 80% of hypertensive patients may be adequately treated with thiazide diuretics *or* beta-adrenergic blocking drugs, *or* both. These two groups are effective and have an acceptably low incidence of side effects.

Thiazide diuretics

Thiazide diuretics lower blood pressure by reducing blood volume and by a direct vasodilator effect. A thiazide such as bendrofluazide (Aprinox) or hydrochlorothiazide (Esidrex, Direma) has a duration of action of at least 24 hours. Only when patients are taking digitalis or develop symptomatic hypokalaemia should either potassium supplements or potassium-sparing agents be given.

Beta-adrenergic blocking drugs

These drugs are now widely used. Beta-blockers inhibit competitively the action of catecholamines on beta-adrenergic receptors. Some block both β_1-receptors (heart rate and force of contraction) and β_2-receptors (vascular and bronchial smooth muscle), whereas others block β_1-receptors, and are relatively cardioselective. They lower blood pressure by reducing cardiac output and by a central effect on the vasomotor centre. They also lower peripheral resistance. There are many beta-blockers available, but those that are cardioselective are preferable in treating hypertension, for example, atenolol (Tenormin) or metoprolol (Betaloc, Lopressor). Many beta-blockers can be given once daily.

Either a thiazide diuretic or a beta-blocker may be used initially in the treatment of hypertension. If one fails to reduce the blood pressure to a desired level the other should be added. When this combination is used the need for potassium supplements is further reduced.

Centrally acting drugs

Methyldopa (Aldomet) has largely been superseded by beta-blockers. However, in those patients who cannot take beta-blockers, methyldopa is the drug of choice. Clonidine (Catapres) is a potent drug, which if withdrawn suddenly is associated with rebound hypertension.

Adrenergic blocking drugs

Guanethidine (Ismelin), bethanidine (Esbatol), and debrisoquine (Declinax) are very potent drugs which produce a gradual fall in peripheral resistance. They have a limited use, however, because of their side effects which include postural hypotension and fluid retention. These drugs have been largely superseded by beta blockers.

Vasodilator drugs

These drugs are used mainly as additional treatment in patients whose conditions are not controlled by thiazides and beta blockers. Hydralazine (Apresoline) is a direct-acting vasodilator that has side effects which can be largely avoided if combined with other drugs. Prazosin (Hypovase) is a potent vasodilator which should be given initially in low dosage, as it occasionally causes severe reduction in blood pressure with associated collapse. Minoxodil (Loniten) and diazoxide (Eudemine) are direct-acting vasodilators with serious side effects and their use is justified only occasionally. Minoxidil causes fluid retention, tachycardia, and hirsutism. Diazoxide causes diabetes, tachycardia, fluid retention and occasionally extrapyramidal central nervous system signs. Nitroprusside (Nipride) can only be given intravenously, and remains the vasodilator for hypertensive crises (especially those associated with left-ventricular failure). (*Swales 1979*)

Other drugs

Spironolactone (Aldactone) is a mild diuretic with potassium-sparing qualities which acts as an aldesterone antagonist. Amiloride (Midamor) and triamterene (Dytac) are potassium-retaining diuretics. Reserpine (Abicol) is a potent drug which has severe side effects, and is now superseded by other drugs. Labetalol (Trandate) is a combined alpha and beta-blocking agent which may be of use in treating patients with obstructive airways disease and left and right heart failure.

NURSING CARE

The nurse's most important role in relation to drug therapy is in patient education. Patient teaching will be considered in greater detail later (p. 254). However, the nurse needs to assess the patient's level of knowledge about his condition and his medications. Effective patient teaching may help compliance in pill-taking. (*Griffith and Madero 1973*)

Patients usually ask questions such as 'What is blood pressure'? and 'What harm does high blood pressure do'? Such questions should be encouraged and not evaded. Verbal information is beneficial, but patients tend to forget soon after, therefore written information in the form of a booklet might be better, as this will reinforce the patient's knowledge. (*Holland 1977*)

The nurse should encourage the patient to get adequate rest and sleep, and to experiment with various behavioural techniques and relaxation procedures such as yoga, transcendental meditation, and biofeedback. Stressful situations should be avoided, and cigarette smoking should be actively discouraged. Regular exercise should be encouraged. Weight reduction may be desired if the patient is obese. Aperients for constipation may be needed, and dietary advice may be helpful. Salt restrictions has little effect on lowering blood pressure, and anyway many patients will have difficulty in complying effectively. Alcohol is a good sedative when used with sense and discretion. Sedatives and hypnotics may be required to ensure adequate rest and minimize anxiety. The nurse should advise that oral contraceptives be discontinued in the presence of hypertension following discussion with medical staff.

Advice on patient's lifestyle

In exceptional cases only, the patient may have to modify his lifestyle, i.e. if he works on high buildings and is receiving anti-hypertensive medication. Patients with malignant hypertension should be told that their condition requires urgent treatment and will necessitate absence from work for a period.

Advice on patients' medication

It is important that patients are given adequate information in order for compliance to be achieved. They should be given verbal and written instruction regarding the frequency and dosage, and any side effects that may be expected to occur. A brief description of the drugs should also be given. They should be encouraged to visit their doctor if side effects occur, and it should be explained that the dosage and frequency may be altered from time to time. It should be ensured that the patient has an up-to-date prescription and an adequate supply of tablets. It should be stressed that the patient may be taking these drugs for the rest of his life, and that he should not stop taking any of them without consulting his doctor. Female patients should also be advised to notify their doctor if they become pregnant.

REFERENCES

Griffith, E.W. & Madero, B. (1973) Primary hypertension: patients' learning needs. *Am. J. Nurs.*, *73*, 624.

Holland, J.M. (1977) *Cardiovascular nursing: prevention, intervention and rehabilitation.* Boston: Little, Brown & Co.

Kannel, W.B. & Dawber, T.R. (1974) Hypertension as an ingredient of a cardiovascular risk profile. *Br. J. hosp. Med.*, *11*, 508.

Richardson, J.F. & Robinson, D. (1971) Variations in the measurement of blood pressure between doctors and nurses. *Jl. R. Col. Gen. Practnr.*, *21*, 698.

Swales, J.D. (1979). *Clinical hypertension.* London: Chapman & Hall Ltd.

9
Rheumatic Fever

Rheumatic fever is a systemic disorder resulting from a cross-sensitivity to a streptococcal infection. The disease is common in Asia, Africa and Eastern Europe, but is becoming progressively less frequent and less severe in many countries, including the United Kingdom and the United States. However, it is more common than is usually realized. Recurrences are frequent unless prophylactic treatment is given. (*Markowitz and Gordis 1972*)

AETIOLOGY

Rheumatic fever in childhood is commonly mild and may be confused with influenza and other viral illnesses. The age of onset is usually between five and twelve years in childhood. In many cases a throat infection with Group A haemolytic streptococci precedes the onset of the disease by 10 to 20 days.

The serum antistreptolysin-O (ASO) titre and erythrocyte sedimentation rate (ESR) are normally raised during the infection and remain high until the onset of the disease. A polymorph leucocytosis is common in the acute stage. A chest X-ray often shows cardiac enlargement, sometimes with a pericardial effusion.

PATHOLOGY

The connective tissues of the myocardium, endocardium and peri-cardium synovial membranes and tendons are in particular affected. The hallmark of rheumatic fever is the Aschoff nodule which may be found in connective tissue of any part of the heart often in close relation to small arterioles. The heart valves may become oedematous. The mitral and aortic valves have small, warty vegetations, consisting of platelets and fibrin. The tricuspid, and very occasionally the pulmonary valves may be involved. Subsequent scarring leads to the valve change of chronic rheumatic heart disease. During the active phase, distortion of the cusps may lead to mitral reflux.

CLINICAL FEATURES

Generally the younger the patient, the more severe is the disease. One or more of the following major clinical features are found.

Carditis
The endocardium, myocardium, and pericardium can all be involved in the rheumatic process. The prime indication of carditis is the appear-ance of significant heart murmurs. Other clinical features are cardio-megaly, heart failure and pericarditis. Active myocarditis is of the utmost importance as it is the main cause of heart failure and death.

Arthritis
This needs to be distinguished from arthralgia. The joint involvement is often migratory. Complete recovery without treatment occurs within three weeks, although the symptoms can be suppressed more rapidly with salicylates or steroids.

ECG changes
Atrioventricular conduction delay can be demonstrated in over 80% of patients with acute rheumatic fever. Apart from prolongation of the P-R interval, prolongation of the Q-T interval may also occur. However, this is difficult to measure.

Chorea
Sydenhams chorea (St Vitus' Dance) is a late manifestation of the rheumatic process, occurring more than two months after the strepto-coccal infection. Chorea is characterized by purposeless involuntary

rapid movements, incoordination and muscle weakness. Speech may be jerky and dribbling occurs. If it is confined to one side it is known as hemichorea. There is no satisfactory treatment, but recovery of normal neurological function occurs, although this may take up to two years.

Erythema marginatum

This is a pink rash which occurs on the trunk and limbs but never the face. It appears superficially similar to the marks left by electrical defibrillation. Other erythematous rashes may also be present.

Subcutaneous nodules

These firm, painless nodules appear over the extensor surfaces of knuckles, elbows, knees, wrists, and over the occiput. They are present for one to six weeks and leave no permanent damage.

Other clinical features include sore throat, malaise and fever. Central chest pain accompanied by fever indicates pericarditis.

TREATMENT

The management of rheumatic fever involves bed rest where there is carditis. However, there is no evidence that prolonged bed rest lessens the incidence of permanent valve damage. Joint immobilization will be required where there is arthritis. Salicylate therapy will also be required. Penicillin therapy and subsequent long-term antibiotic prophylaxis should be given. Steroids are only of use in selected patients.

Heart failure is treated with digoxin and diuretics in the usual way. Pericardial effusions may require therapeutic aspiration.

Convalescence in a suitable environment will be required when the active stage is over and before return to school or work. (*Doyle 1974*)

PROGNOSIS

A complete recovery takes place in the vast majority of patients. However, a recurrence of rheumatic fever is common during childhood and early adult life. Sixty percent of patients who have had rheumatic fever develop subsequent valve disease. The more severe forms and multiple valve lesions occur after recurrent attacks of rheumatic fever.

The commonest lesions are mitral stenosis and incompetence, both of which are more common in females. Aortic valve disease is more frequently seen in men. Tricuspid and pulmonary valve disease are much less commonly involved. Other sequelae may occur, e.g. rheumatic cardiomyopathy.

REFERENCES

Doyle, E. (1974) Rheumatic fever: a continuing problem. *Cardiovasc. Nurs.*, *10*, 17.
Markowitz, N. & Gordis, L. (1972) *Rheumatic fever*. Philadelphia: Saunders.

10
Diseases of the Valves

MITRAL STENOSIS

AETIOLOGY

Mitral stenosis is almost invariably due to rheumatic fever. Congenital mitral stenosis is an uncommon condition. The disease is four times as frequent in females as in males.

The incidence approximately parallels that of acute rheumatic fever. It is much commoner in the Middle East, the Tropics and the Indian Sub-Continent.

PATHOLOGY

Narrowing of the valve occurs by fusion of the cusps at the points of insertion of the shortest chordae tendinae. This usually gives rise to a funnel-shaped deformity of the valve with a button-hole orifice. This narrowing is a slow, progressive process due to the deposition of platelets and fibrin. There are no symptoms until the valve area has been reduced to 2.5 cm^2 (the normal area is 5 cm^2). The symptoms are usually severe when the valve area is less than 1 cm^2.

The left ventricle is usually normal or small in size in pure mitral stenosis, but occasionally considerable ventricular dilatation may occur. Elevation of the left atrial, pulmonary venous, and pulmonary pressures is followed by interstitial fibrosis of the lungs and thickening of the alveolar walls, so that the lungs become abnormally stiff. There is medial hypertrophy and intimal fibrosis of the small pulmonary arteries, which may extend to the arterioles. The main pulmonary arteries may also show atheroma associated with pulmonary hypertension which causes right ventricular and right atrial hypertrophy. This persistently raised right heart pressure causes chronic congestion of the liver and cardiac cirrhosis.

HAEMODYNAMICS

Narrowing of the mitral valve leads to elevation of the left atrial pressure (LAP). At first this occurs only during atrial systole. If the narrowing increases there is a pressure gradient throughout diastole; the pulmonary venous and pulmonary capillary pressure rise causing vascular engorgement and increased stiffness of the lung. At the same time the pulmonary artery pressure rises passively to maintain the usual pressure difference between the pulmonary artery and the pulmonary vein and ensure a normal blood flow. Acute pulmonary oedema will occur if the mean LAP exceeds 30 mmHg.

AGGRAVATING FACTORS

Patients may become severely symptomatic as a result of:

1. Intercurrent chest infections.
2. Pulmonary emboli.
3. Atrial fibrillation with a rapid ventricular rate.
4. Thyrotoxicosis.
5. Pregnancy, either in the first trimester as cardiac output rises, at term, or at delivery.

CLINICAL FEATURES

There is usually a long, silent interval of about 10 – 20 years between rheumatic fever and the development of symptoms.

Dyspnoea
At first this may occur on exertion, caused by decreased pulmonary compliance because of the interstitial oedema. Eventually orthopnoea develops.

Bronchitis

Recurrent bronchitis often associated with wheezing, results from mucosal oedema caused by congestion of the bronchial veins which drain to the pulmonary venous system. This symptom usually occurs in winter.

Haemoptysis

It is not unusual for haemoptysis to present as the first symptom of the disease, though this is seldom severe. It may result from a chest infection, pulmonary infarction, or acute pulmonary oedema.

Patients with the complications of pulmonary hypertension or atrial fibrillation develop right heart failure with fatigue, oedema, and hepatic pain, especially if there is tricuspid incompetence. These symptoms may be mistaken for angina. True angina is seldom seen with severe pulmonary hypertension.

Mitral facies

If the cardiac output is low, peripheral vasoconstriction in the skin leads to pallor and cyanosis of the blush area, producing a malar flush.

Pulses

The volume of the aterial pulse is reduced in proportion to the severity of the stenosis. Atrial fibrillation is common. The jugular venous pulse is usually normal but prominent 'a' waves occur with pulmonary hypertension.

Apex beat

This is usually in the normal place but may be deviated to the left by right ventricular hypertrophy. The cardiac impulse is classically described as 'tapping' and this is because of a palpable loud first heart sound.

Auscultation

There are four classical auscultatory signs of mitral stenosis: a loud *first heart sound* (it may be so loud that it can be felt), an *opening snap* (due to the movements of the valve cusps being suddenly stopped because they are stuck together), a *mid-systolic murmur* caused by obstruction of blood flow through the valve which cannot open properly), and a *pre-systolic murmur* (due to the propulsion of blood through the mitral valve by atrial systole). The pre-systolic murmur disappears with the onset of atrial fibrillation. As the mitral valve becomes more calcified and less mobile, the first sound and the opening snap may disappear.

COMPLICATIONS

Atrial fibrillation

Atrial fibrillation (AF) is an important complication which develops in a large proportion of cases of mitral stenosis. It is almost invariable in patients over the age of forty. At its onset the ventricular rate of AF is often more than 140 per minute which may precipitate acute pulmonary oedema. AF in mitral stenosis is responsible for the development of systemic emboli, which may occur in a few days. Some 20% of mitral patients have an embolus during their lives. It is not uncommon for functional tricuspid incompetence and right heart failure to follow AF.

Pulmonary hypertension

About 20% of patients demonstrate an unexplained reactive pulmonary hypertension.

Subacute bacterial endocarditis

This is relatively infrequent in mitral stenosis.

INVESTIGATIONS

The ECG may show a bifid P wave, indicating left atrial enlargement. AF is common. Evidence of right ventricular hypertrophy develops in cases with severe pulmonary hypertension.

The chest X-ray may show evidence of left atrial hypertrophy, pulmonary venous congestion, and even mitral valve calcification. Pulmonary artery, right ventricular and, occasionally, right atrial enlargement may also be present if there is pulmonary arterial hypertension. The echocardiogram provides the best information of diagnostic value, and a rough guide to the severity of the lesion.

Cardiac catheterization is not usually necessary, but may still be performed in atypical cases, or where adequate echocardiography is not available. If a satisfactory pulmonary capillary wedge pressure (PWP) cannot be obtained by right heart catheterization, an accurate measurement of the pressure gradient across the mitral valve can be obtained by a direct puncture of the left atrium by the trans-septal approach.

TREATMENT

Medical treatment

Mild stenosis causes no disability and no treatment is required. These patients should be encouraged to lead reasonably normal lives, but to avoid excessive exertion. Mild dyspnoea usually responds to treatment with diuretics, whilst AF should be treated with digoxin to control the rapid ventricular rate. Anticoagulant therapy should be given to reduce the risk of systemic embolism to all patients with AF. Chest infections should be treated with appropriate antibiotics. In patients younger than 21 years of age, penicillin should be given prophylactically against further attacks of rheumatic fever. In all patients with heart valve disease, prophylactic antibiotics should be given for dental extractions to prevent bacterial endocarditis.

Surgical treatment

If mitral stenosis causes mechanical obstruction to the circulation, then surgery is probably required. There are two types of surgery available: mitral valvotomy and mitral valve replacement.

Mitral valvotomy gives good results when the valve is pliant. The criteria for selecting patients for valvotomy are:

1. Symptoms must be significant.
2. Valve must be mobile.
3. Absence of mitral incompetence.
4. No calcium in the valve visible on X-ray.
5. Mobile, thin cusps on echocardiogram.

If the above are present, mitral valve replacement may be required, which involves cardiopumonary bypass facilities. The commonest type of prosthetic valve used is the Starr-Edwards caged ball device. (*Harken 1974*)

In mitral valvotomy two methods can be used. The *closed mitral valvotomy* is the classical method for uncomplicated cases. A dilator is introduced through the apex of the beating left ventricle under the control of a finger in the left atrium through the mitral valve. The dilator is then opened, thus opening up the mitral valve orifice. The *open mitral valvotomy* method is used whenever a thrombus in the left atrium is strongly suspected.

PROGNOSIS

Patients with severe mitral stenosis become completely incapacitated from dyspnoea, which is usually the first complaint. In the majority of patients some complications arise. Once right heart failure has developed, the prognosis without surgical intervention is poor. The average life expectation from the onset of symptoms is about 10 years.

MITRAL INCOMPETENCE (synonyms: mitral insufficiency, regurgitation, reflux)

AETIOLOGY

Mitral incompetence is usually the result of previous rheumatic valvulitis. Other 'non-rheumatic' causes, whereby the mitral valve cusps, chordae tendinae, papillary muscles or valve ring may be affected, are:

Congenital
Subacute bacterial endocarditis (SBE)
Mitral valve prolapse
Papillary muscle dysfunction
Chordal rupture
Hypertrophic obstructive cardiomyopathy (HOCM)
Left ventricular dilatation
Endomyocardial fibrosis

Mitral incompetence, unlike stenosis, is more common in males.

PATHOLOGY

The mitral valve ring often dilates and the cusps are unable to close the enlarged orifice. The valve cusps and chordae become scarred and retract over a period of years, so that although the valve ring may return to normal, the cusps are too small to close the normal sized orifice, and the fibrosed chordae and papillary muscles interfere with the valve closing mechanism. Eventually the incompetent valve is rigid and calcification is present.

HAEMODYNAMICS

The process just described occurs over a period of years. Pure mitral incompetence is associated with a large increase in left ventricular output. Since the pressure in the left atrium is lower than that in the aorta, the resistance to left ventricular ejection is reduced and the stroke volume may be increased up to three times normal.

The left atrium is allowed to dilate, thus accommodating the regurgitant stream of blood without a significant rise in left atrial pressure. Later the left ventricle may dilate and may eventually fail. In acute myocardial infarction, regurgitation of blood into a stiff left atrium produces a sudden increase in pulmonary venous pressure, and acute pulmonary oedema. The effect on pulmonary venous, capillary and arterial pressures is not as great as in mitral stenosis, and right ventricular hypertrophy is less marked.

PROGNOSIS

This depends upon the severity of mitral incompetence. In mild cases pulmonary congestion is less impressive than in mitral stenosis, but the risk of SBE is greater, and a few patients may die suddenly. Acute mitral incompetence due to rupture of the chordae or papillary muscles may be rapidly fatal. If they do not respond to medical treatment with digoxin and diuretics, then mitral valve replacement helps dramatically.

CLINICAL FEATURES

The symptoms depend on how suddenly the regurgitation develops.

Dyspnoea
This occurs on exertion. Fatigue usually ensues.

Heart failure
Right heart failure may follow left ventricular failure rapidly when induced by atrial fibrillation.

Pulses
The arterial pulse is often of small volume. Atrial fibrillation is common in older patients. The venous pressure is normal unless severe pulmonary hypertension is present.

Apex beat
The cardiac impulse is displaced to the left. A systolic thrill may be felt.

Auscultation

The *first heart sound* is soft and followed by a full-length *systolic murmur*. The *second heart sound* may be split. A *third heart sound* is heard which is caused by rapid ventricular filling.

INVESTIGATIONS

The ECG may show broad and bifid P waves indicating left atrial enlargement. AF is common. Left ventricular hypertrophy is also seen; the QRS voltage is therefore increased.

The chest X-ray may show evidence of left atrial or ventricular hypertrophy. The valve ring may be calcified. Pulmonary changes may be present depending on the pulmonary venous and arterial pressures.

The mitral valve echocardiogram may be abnormal, showing prolapse with cusp remnants visible in the left atrium during systole.

Cardiac catheterization and cine-angiography are not usually necessary when the clinical and echocardiographic findings are typical. The usual findings are increased left heart pressure. Increased right heart pressure may also be present. Left ventricular cardio-angiography demonstrates the presence of mitral incompetence by reflux of a dye back into the left atrium from the dilated left ventricle.

TREATMENT

This depends upon the degree and type of incompetence involved. Acute mitral incompetence may require emergency valve replacement. Antibiotic prophylaxis against SBE is indicated before dental treatment and other minor procedures producing bacteraemia. Routine anticoagulation may be given to patients with AF.

AORTIC STENOSIS

AETIOLOGY

Aortic stenosis occurs in about one quarter of all patients with chronic valvular heart disease. About 80% of these cases are male. There are three causes:

Congenital
Rheumatic
Degenerative changes

PATHOLOGY

The pathology depends on the aetiology. In *congenital* cases the valve is often bicuspid and becomes heavily calcified in adult life. In *rheumatic* cases there is adhesion at the commisures and the cusps are fibrotic, shrunken, calcified and leaky. In *senile* cases the cusps are grossly calcified thereby reducing mobility. Irrespective of aetiology, there is almost always some calcification by the age of forty years.

HAEMODYNAMICS

Haemodynamic consequences occur as soon as the orifice area is reduced to about 50%. The primary abnormality is obstruction to left ventricular outflow which leads to a pressure gradient between the left ventricle and aorta during systole. The left ventricle hypertrophies and later dilates. The end-diastolic pressure in the left ventricle increases causing a rise in left atrial pressure also. Pulmonary congestion may then appear.

Calcification of the valve may also involve the coronary ostia causing impaired inflow to the coronary arteries. Even if the vessels are unaffected, relative coronary insufficiency is common owing to discrepancies between the needs of the hypertrophied myocardium and the coronary flow. Blood is ejected through the stenosed aortic valve in a jet which hits the aortic wall and produces a dilatation of the ascending aorta.

CLINICAL FEATURES

Most patients have gradually increasing obstruction for years but do not become symptomatic until the fourth or fifth decade.

Angina pectoris

A common feature in spite of essentially normal coronary vessels in a large proportion of the patients.

Dyspnoea

Starts as dyspnoea on exertion and may progress to orthopnoea and even pulmonary oedema. It is a sign of left ventricular failure.

Syncope on effort

Regarded as an ominous symptom of aortic stenosis. It may be caused by a fall in blood pressure during exertion or by transient attacks of ventricular fibrillation or asystole.

Dizziness

Most frequent when standing. Probably due to low arterial blood pressure and orthostatic mechanisms.

Palpation

Reveals a powerful thrust in the apical region. A systolic thrill may be felt at the base of the heart and along the carotid arteries.

Auscultation

A mid-systolic murmur is usually found at the second right interspace. Opening of the valve may produce an ejection click.

INVESTIGATIONS

The ECG usually shows sinus rhythm. It may show left ventricular hypertrophy and strain.

The chest X-Ray is often helpful in detecting calcification of the aortic valve. The heart is often of normal size, but with a rounded left contour as a sign of LVH. The ascending aorta is usually prominent owing to post-stenotic dilatation. As heart failure develops the heart size increases and signs of pulmonary congestion appear in the lung fields.

The phonocardiogram shows a 'diamond-shaped', crescendo-decrescendo systolic murmur. The echocardiogram shows thickening of the left ventricular wall. Cardiac catheterization indicates the severity of the stenosis, which is estimated from the systolic pressure gradient between the left ventricle and the aorta and the simultaneous flow across the aortic orifice. Cine-angiography is used to visualize the anatomy of the stenosed valve and the contractile pattern of the myocardium.

TREATMENT

Surgical treatment by valve replacement is the only hope of relief of the obstruction. The mortality of the operation is 6 – 10%, and so surgery should not be performed uncritically. The medical treatment consists of advice in avoiding strenuous physical activity, to treat the heart failure, and to deal with the angina pectoris.

PROGNOSIS

This is poor if treated medically, but is radically improved by surgical intervention. Cases of mild aortic stenosis have a good prognosis if there is no appreciable degree of LVH, and can be expected to live twenty to fifty years.

AORTIC INCOMPETENCE (synonyms: aortic insufficiency, regurgitation, reflux)

AETIOLOGY

Three quarters of all patients with pure or predominant incompetence are males. However, females predominate among patients with aortic incompetence who have associated mitral disease.

Rheumatic fever is still considered the most common cause of aortic incompetence. Other causes include:

Syphilis
Subacute bacterial endocarditis (SBE)
Marfans syndrome
Ankylosing spondylitis
Reiters syndrome
Hypertension

Congenital aortic incompetence is very uncommon but congenital defects may predispose to bacterial endocarditis, with subsequent severe valve incompetence.

PATHOLOGY

In rheumatic cases there is fibrosis, shrinkage and distortion of the cusps causing incompetence but as the commisures are also adherent some associated stenosis is common. In syphilis there is widening of the commisures and dilatation of the aorta and aortic valve ring. In severe hypertension, dilatation of the aorta may lead to slight aortic valve incompetence but the cusps are usually normal and there is no stenosis.

HAEMODYNAMICS

The total stroke volume expelled by the left ventricle is increased by aortic incompetence. Left ventricular function deteriorates and the end-diastolic pressure increases. The left ventricle therefore dilates and, later, hypertrophies. A rise in left atrial pressure and the development of pulmonary congestion ensue. Myocardial ischaemia occurs because both left ventricular dilatation and the elevated left ventricular systolic pressure tend to augment myocardial oxygen requirements.

CLINICAL FEATURES

About one third of patients with aortic valve incompetence are reported to have symptoms which are considered as 'functional' rather than as signs of the severity of the disease.

Palpitations
Often most distressing on lying down. Sinus tachycardia occurring during exertion or with emotion may produce particularly uncomfortable palpitations, as well as head pounding. These complaints may persist for many years before the development of exertional dyspnoea.

Dyspnoea
Appears when the left ventricle fails. It is followed by orthopnoea, and paroxysmal nocturnal dyspnoea.

Angina pectoris
Less common in aortic incompetence than stenosis.

Pulses
The large pulse amplitude often produces a 'water-hammer' or collapsing pulse as a result of the sharp pressure rise followed by an equally rapid fall in pressure from the retrograde flow of blood through the incompetent valve. 'Corrigans sign' (exaggerated pulsation in the neck) is also present.

Apex beat
This is displaced to the left and downwards as a sign of left ventricular dilatation. A powerful systolic thrust in the apex region may be felt.

Auscultation
A high-pitched diastolic murmur starting at the second heart sound is heard. There is frequently a mid-systolic murmur in the same position (left sternal border). In severe cases a pre-systolic or delayed diastolic murmur resembling that of mitral stenosis may be heard at the apex (Austin Flint murmur).

INVESTIGATIONS

The phonocardiogram shows the diastolic murmur as a diminuendo-shape. The systolic murmur is characteristically 'diamond-shaped'. The ECG may be fairly normal for many years. However, as the severity of aortic incompetence increases the ECG shows signs of left ventricular hypertrophy. The chest X-Ray usually shows an increased heart size caused by left ventricular enlargement. In heart failure signs of pulmonary congestion may be seen in the lung fields. Occasionally valvular calcifications may occur. The echocardiogram often shows a vibration of the anterior leaflet of the mitral valve, and, if the regurgitation is severe, the mitral valve is seen to close abnormally early. Cardiac catheterization and cine-angiography is necessary when the degree of severity is in doubt.

TREATMENT

This depends partly on the aetiology and partly on the severity of the lesion. Thus patients with endocarditis require treatment with the appropriate antibiotics. Syphilis should be treated with penicillin. Digitalis and diuretics will be required for left ventricular failure, and drugs for any apparent angina. If the aortic incompetence is severe, aortic valve replacement will be necessary, either with a prosthetic or homograft valve.

PROGNOSIS

The natural history or aortic incompetence depends on the aetiology, the severity and the rate of development. Patients with chronic rheumatic incompetence may remain in a compensated state for many years. However, if the lesion is severe, gradual deterioration is common. If there is a sudden increase (as in bacterial endocarditis) rapid deterioration may occur.

TRICUSPID STENOSIS

AETIOLOGY

Tricuspid stenosis is generally part of complex rheumatic heart disease. Rare causes include:

Carcinoid tumours
Systemic lupus erythematosus (SLE)
Congenital tricuspid stenosis

PATHOLOGY

When the lesion is due to rheumatic heart disease, the pathological appearance is similar to that of mitral valve disease. The valve cusps are thickened and the chordae may be adherent and shortened. Some degree of incompetence is present. The right atrium is dilated and hypertrophied, and the venae cavae are also dilated. There is usually cardiac cirrhosis of the liver.

HAEMODYNAMICS

Narrowing of the tricuspid valve obstructs blood flow from the right atrium to the ventricle during ventricular diastole. This causes an abnormally high right atrial pressure, and a fall in the cardiac output due to the increased resistance to blood flow. Atrial fibrillation is often present.

CLINICAL FEATURES

In most cases of tricuspid stenosis, mitral stenosis is also present and dominates the clinical picture.

Dyspnoea
This is due to the presence of mitral stenosis

Jugular pulse
Large 'a' waves are produced in sinus rhythm, but disappear in atrial fibrillation.

Auscultation
Mid-diastolic and pre-systolic murmurs may be heard at the lower left sternal edge. They are accentuated on inspiration, because of increased return to the right atrium.

INVESTIGATIONS

The ECG shows tall P waves indicating right atrial enlargement. The

P-R interval is often prolonged. The chest X-Ray demonstrates a large atrium with the features of associated mitral valve disease. The echocardiogram may reveal delayed closure of the valve which is situated anterior to the mitral valve. Cardiac catheterization demonstrates a diastolic pressure difference between the right atrium and ventricle.

TREATMENT

Surgery is normally only undertaken if the stenosis is responsible for major symptoms. Appropriate surgical treatment of the mitral and aortic valves may need to be considered as well as replacement of the tricuspid valve. Medical treatment of severe stenosis is unsatisfactory.

PROGNOSIS

Rheumatic tricuspid valve disease is invariably associated with serious mitral disease and often with aortic valve disease as well. Following surgical treatment the prognosis is relatively good.

TRICUSPID INCOMPETENCE (synonyms: tricuspid regurgitation, reflux)

AETIOLOGY

Tricuspid incompetence may be functional (no disease of the valve leaflets) or organic. More often it is functional. Functional tricuspid incompetence is a common complication of right ventricular failure and pulmonary hypertension. Organic tricuspid incompetence may be:

Congenital — Ebstein's anomaly (downward displacement of abnormally formed tricuspid valve ring and leaflets into the right ventricle).
Endocardial cushion defects.
Acquired — Traumatic (may follow blunt injury).
Bacterial endocarditis.
Rheumatic: seen in association with mitral valve disease.

PATHOLOGY

In functional tricuspid incompetence the valve ring is greatly dilated and the cusps are not big enough to close the enlarged orifice. In cases due to organic rheumatic disease, the cusps are fibrosed and distorted with some associated stenosis. The right atrium and ventricle are dilated and hypertrophied and there is hepatic congestion.

HAEMODYNAMICS

The incompetent valve allows blood to flow into the right atrium during ventricular systole. Consequently there is a systolic rise of pressure in the right atrium which is transmitted to the jugular and hepatic veins which produce a characteristic large systolic ('cv') wave. Both diastolic and systolic flow through the valve is increased on inspiration as an increased volume of blood is drawn into the heart.

CLINICAL FEATURES

Co-existent mitral valve disease often dominates the clinical picture.

Dyspnoea
This and orthopnoea are the major symptoms, although orthopnoea may disappear.

Oedema
This and ascites may occur as the disease progresses. Hepatic enlargement is also often present.

Jugular pulse
A large systolic wave is present in the jugular veins and sometimes over the liver.

Auscultation
A systolic murmur is heard at the lower left sternal edge which is usually increased on inspiration.

INVESTIGATIONS

The ECG usually shows AF with right ventricular hypertrophy. The chest X-Ray usually shows right atrial enlargement. Cardiac catherterization and cine-angiography show the large systolic venous wave of the right atrial pulse. The finding of severe pulmonary hypertension indicates that the incompetence is functional, whereas a relatively normal pulmonary artery pressure indicates organic incompetence. The echocardiogram of functional tricuspid incompetence shows that the amplitude of valve movement is increased although the closure rate is normal.

TREATMENT

When the clinical features are mild, no specific treatment is required. Digitalis and diuretic therapy often have a striking effect. Maintenance anticoagulant therapy (to reduce the risk of pulmonary and systemic embolism) are indicated if AF develops.

Organic tricuspid incompetence may require valve replacement.

PROGNOSIS

This depends on the severity and treatment. The disease is often tolerated for a long time, although 70% of patients die before the age of 55 years.

PULMONARY STENOSIS

AETIOLOGY

Pulmonary stenosis is usually of congenital origin; acquired stenosis is extremely rare, but causes include:

Rheumatic heart disease
Carcinoid syndrome
Hypertrophic cardiomyopathy

Pulmonary stenosis comprises approximately 10% of all congenital heart disease.

PATHOLOGY

The valve is usually tricuspid and the valve cusps are fused along their margins to form an obstructing diaphragm. In mild cases, the hole in the diaphragm may be only 5 – 10 mm in diameter as compared to a normal valve opening of 5 cm. In severe cases it may be no more than 2 – 3 mm in diameter. The pulmonary artery is dilated and the right ventricle is hypertrophied.

HAEMODYNAMICS

There is a pressure difference between the right ventricle and the main pulmonary artery during right ventricular systole, resulting in a high right ventricular systolic pressure with a normal or low pulmonary arterial pressure. The duration of ventricular systole is prolonged in order to compensate for the effects of the obstruction.

CLINICAL FEATURES

In a substantial proportion of patients with pulmonary stenosis, the lesion is so mild that symptoms never occur.

Pulses

The arterial pulse is usually normal. The venous pulse is also usually normal, but if the lesion is severe the 'a' wave is increased as the force of right atrial contraction is increased to compensate for the stiff right ventricle.

Palpation

There is nearly always a systolic thrill in the second left intercostal space.

Auscultation

The first heart sound is normal, but it is often followed by an early systolic 'ejection' click and a loud mid-systolic murmur best heard in the second left intercostal space.

Dyspnoea

This may present, especially on effort. Syncope and angina may also present.

INVESTIGATIONS

The ECG provides evidence of the severity of the stenosis, e.g. in general, the greater the degree of right ventricular hypertrophy, the tighter the stenosis. Right axis deviation and right atrial hypertrophy are common features. The chest X-ray may demonstrate dilatation of the main and often the left pulmonary artery. Cardiac enlargement is not to be expected. Cardiac catheterization provides confirmatory evidence.

TREATMENT

If the lesion is severe the patient's activities will be limited by increasing fatigue and breathlessness. Right heart failure may supervene in middle life. Pulmonary valve replacement is recommended for patients with moderate or severe stenosis.

PROGNOSIS

The infant with severe pulmonary stenosis may be critically ill and require urgent surgical relief. If the stenosis is mild, a normal or nearly normal life span is to be expected.

PULMONARY INCOMPETENCE (synonyms: pulmonary insufficiency, regurgitation, reflux)

AETIOLOGY

Pulmonary incompetence is usually secondary to pulmonary hypertension. Other causes are:

Bacterial endocarditis
Congenital

It is nearly always overshadowed by the heart disease to which it is secondary.

HAEMODYNAMICS

Pulmonary incompetence does not produce any serious haemodynamic effects. The lesions causing severe incompetence undoubtedly increase the volume load of the right ventricle. The heart enlarges and the right ventricular volume and systolic pressure rise, but the diastolic pressure is little changed.

CLINICAL FEATURES

In most cases there are signs of pulmonary hypertension.

Auscultation

The only feature which suggests pulmonary incompetence is an early diastolic murmur (Graham Steell murmur) in the second or third left intercostal spaces which becomes louder on inspiration. It is difficult to distinguish it from that of aortic incompetence.

INVESTIGATIONS

Cardiac catheterization and cine-angiography will confirm the diagnosis.

TREATMENT

Relief of pulmonary hypertension, when possible, abolishes the leak. Surgical intervention is not indicated for the incompetence itself.

PROGNOSIS

Pulmonary incompetence does not appreciably alter the prognosis of pulmonary hypertensive disease.

REFERENCE

Harken, D.E. (1974) Post-operative care following heart valve surgery. *Heart & Lung, 3*, 893.

11
Diseases of the Pericardium, Myocardium, and Endocardium

PERICARDIUM

NORMAL FUNCTION

The visceral pericardium is a serous membrane, separated by a small amount of fluid from a fibrous sac, the parietal pericardium. The pericardium prevents sudden dilatation of the cardiac chambers during exercise and hypervolaemia. It holds the heart in a fixed position, minimizes friction between the heart and surrounding structures, prevents displacement of the heart, and kinking of the great vessels. It also probably retards the spread of infections from the lungs and pleural cavities to the heart.

The main disorders affecting the pericardium fall into three groups:

Pericarditis
Constriction of tamponade
Pericardial effusion

PERICARDITIS

Aetiology
Causes of pericarditis include:

Acute idiopathic or nonspecific (probably viral)
Infections: bacterial, viral, tuberculous and fungal
Acute myocardial infarction
Malignancy
Post-myocardial and post-cardiotomy syndromes
Rheumatic fever
Trauma
Drugs, i.e. procainamide (Pronestyl), hydralazine (Apresoline) and practolol (Eraldin)

Pathology
Fibrinous inflammation with little effusion is often apt to occur. Adhesions between the visceral and parietal surfaces also occur.

Clinical features
Pain. This is often severe. It is usually pleuritic, but may be over-shadowed by the constrictive pain resembling that of myocardial ischaemia. The pain may be felt either in the precordium or in one or both of the shoulders. It may be aggravated by coughing, swallowing, inspiration, lying flat or on rotation of the trunk. It is often relieved by sitting up and leaning forward.

Pericardial friction rub. This is the cardinal physical sign. It is heard most frequently during forced expiration, with the patient leaning forward. It is usually a scratchy or grating noise, heard in systole, mid-diastole and pre-systole, or in only one of these phases. It is often localized to a small area but varies in position from time to time. The rub is heard most commonly along the left sternal edge.

Investigations
ECG. This usually displays widespread elevation of the ST segments (with the ST segment concave upwards), without significant changes in the QRS complexes. Several days later, the ST segments return to normal and the T waves then become inverted. The ECG may simulate that of acute myocardial infarction, but Q waves are not seen, the ST segment elevation is of different configuration, and the T wave inversion occurs only after return of the ST segment to the iso-electric line.

Sinus tachycardia often seems to occur during the early development of pericarditis.

Chest X-ray. This shows a normal heart outline unless there is an associated effusion.

Treatment

Specific treatment depends on the aetiology of the pericarditis. All patients with acute pericarditis should be observed frequently and carefully for the possibility of a developing effusion or, if this is already present, for signs of tamponade.

Treatment generally consists of pain relief, the removal of fluid when this is causing tamponade, and the treatment of the underlying cause when this is possible.

PERICARDIAL EFFUSION

This consists of an accumulation of fluid in the pericardial sac which may accompany acute pericarditis or occur in a variety of chronic conditions.

Clinical features

Pericardial effusion is especially important when it develops within a relatively short time. The pericardium becomes taut and filling of the heart is impaired, especially when the pericardial tension is further increased by inspiration.

Pulses. The venous pressure may rise and the arterial pulse volume diminish in inspiration. This is called a *paradoxical venous pulse* since it is the reverse of normal.

Percussion. Large effusions may be detected by percussion. With the patient lying flat, increased dullness may be noted in the second left interspace, and to the left of the apex beat.

Auscultation. This may reveal pericardial friction and heart sounds which are often soft.

Investigations.

Chest X-ray. Differentiation from heart enlargement may be difficult. Fluoroscopy may be more helpful.

Echocardiogram. This is undoubtedly the most reliable non-invasive investigation. An echo-free zone can be seen in front of the right ventricle and behind the left ventricle.

ECG. Pericardial effusion produces low voltage ECG complexes which may vary in amplitude from cycle to cycle (electrical alternans).

Treatment

The specific cause of the effusion should be found and treated wherever possible. Where an effusion has been diagnosed but there are no significant haemodynamic changes, there is no indication for immediate pericardial aspiration. If, however, any signs of deterioration occur such as:

Tachycardia
Elevated JVP
Decreased blood pressure

then the patient should be thoroughly examined, and aspiration needs to be seriously considered.

Pericardial aspiration

A lumbar puncture is usually suitable for this procedure. Two approaches are used: xiphisternal and precordial. The patient should be in a semi-reclining position with the thorax at an angle of between $45°$ and $60°$ to the horizontal.

In most cases it is sufficient to withdraw a small quantity of fluid for the necessary laboratory investigations. If an evacuating procedure is necessary, the needle should be fixed in a position near the outside border of the pericardial sac.

HAEMOPERICARDIUM

Although any pericardial effusion may contain some blood, it is quite rare for the fluid haematocrit to exceed 10%. In some cases, however, the pericardium may become filled with pure blood following haemorrhage. This may occur due to:

Trauma of the thorax.
Rupture of the ventricle in transmural myocardial infarction.
Rupture of an aortic dissection.
Tear of the right ventricle during pericardial puncture.
Malignant effusion.

The evolution of these cases is nearly always dramatic, with the rapid development of cardiac tamponade.

CARDIAC TAMPONADE (PERICARDIAL TAMPONDAE)

This is the accumulation of fluid in the pericardium in an amount sufficient to cause serious obstruction to the inflow of blood to the ventricles. The amount of fluid necessary to produce this state may be as small as 250 ml or as large as one litre.

Tamponade results most often from bleeding into the pericardial space following cardiac surgery, trauma (including cardiac perforation during diagnostic procedures), tuberculosis, pyogenic infection, or malignancy, but it may occur in acute viral or idiopathic pericarditis and haemopericardium which may result when a patient with any form of acute pericarditis is treated with anticoagulants.

The inability of the ventricles to fill during diastole, leads to raised diastolic pressures in the ventricles, an increase in systemic and pulmonary venous pressures, and a fall in cardiac output and blood pressure. There is a compensatory sinus tachycardia and the pulse is often described as being of the paradoxical type.

CONSTRICTIVE PERICARDITIS

Aetiology
The aetiology of constrictive pericarditis is usually infectious, either tuberculous or viral. Other causes include:

Fungal infections.
Parasitic infections.
Rheumatoid arthritis.
Radiation.

Pathology
The heart is encased in dense fibrous tissue which may be calcified. The epicardium may also be thickened so that there is a constrictive epicarditis.

Haemodynamics
The basic abnormality is the inability of the ventricles to fill adequately during diastole because of the limitations imposed by the rigid, thickened pericardium. Because filling is restricted, the venous pressure is therefore

high. The stroke volume is low and there is a compensatory tachycardia.

Clinical features

The features are predominantly those of right heart failure. The presenting feature is that of fatigue and dyspnoea on effort.

Pulses. The pulse is of small volume and may be 'paradoxical'. The venous pressure is high and the pulse shows an abrupt but shallow 'Y' descent. Sinus tachycardia and later atrial fibrillation often occur.

Auscultation. A high pitched early third heart sound may be heard due to rapid ventricular filling.

Palpation. There may be a palpable early diastolic thrust over the heart which occurs at the same time as the third heart sound.

There may be pronounced ascites, oedema and hepatomegaly.

Investigations

Chest X-ray. The heart is usually small or normal in size, but may be occasionally enlarged due to thickening of the pericardium. Calcification may also be seen. Reduced cardiac pulsation is seen on fluoroscopy.

ECG. There are low-voltage QRS complexes associated with flattened or slightly inverted T waves. The P waves may be large or bifid if AF is not present.

Cardiac catheterization. This reveals a normal or slightly reduced cardiac output at rest, and an increased filling pressure. The ventricular pressure shows a dip-plateau pattern during diastole. However, this appearance also occurs in cardiomyopathy.

Treatment:

Surgical intervention is always required. Following this almost normal haemodynamics can be expected, although the full benefits may not be apparent until several months later. (*Hirschmann 1978*)

Prognosis

Following surgical intervention the prognosis is usually quite good. However, if these has been extensive myocardial involvement or severe liver damage, the outlook may not be so good.

MYOCARDIUM

The myocardium is involved in most types of heart disease. Direct impairment of myocardial function occurs in two ways. Firstly, the myocardium itself may be affected by disease, or secondly, its effective working may be embarrassed by disease of the pericardium or, more rarely, the endocardium.

The most common myocardial disease is ischaemic disease resulting from atheroma of the coronary arteries. Infarction or diffuse fibrosis reduces the contractile power of the ventricles. Other types of myocardial diseases are usually attributed to congenital or valve disease, thyrotoxicosis or hypertension.

Two relatively uncommon types of myocardial disease, myocarditis and cardiomyopathy, will be considered here.

MYOCARDITIS

This is an acute or chronic inflammation of the myocardium due to infective or toxic agents or by abnormal immunological responses.

Aetiology

Infectious — viral, rickettsial or bacterial.
Parasitic — as in trichinosis or toxoplasmosis.
Immune disorders.
Connective tissue disorders.
Acute rheumatic fever.

Clinical features
Dyspnoea. This is the main symptom, and may be followed by the development of right and left heart failure.

Precordial discomfort. This may be more marked if pericarditis is associated with the myocarditis. Ischaemic heart disease may be misdiagnosed when there is precordial discomfort and dyspnoea associated with ST changes on the ECG.

Investigations
ECG. Mild forms of myocarditis may cause only sinus tachycardia and non-specific changes. They may also give rise to arrhythmias such as

atrial fibrillation, paroxysmal atrial tachycardia and conduction disturbances. In severe cases there may be ventricular ectopic beats, tachyarrhythmias or a bradycardia due to heart block. These arrhythmias
may be responsible for sudden death. Occasionally, there is ST elevation
or depression, or inversion of T waves.

Chest X-ray. This shows cardiomegaly with pulmonary congestion or
oedema.

Echocardiogram. This will exclude a large pericardial effusion, mitral
stenosis as a cause of heart failure and confirm poor left ventricular
function.

Cardiac biopsy. This may be performed in the acute phase in order to
obtain a histological diagnosis and attempt to detect virus antibody or
virus particles.

Treatment
There is no specific treatment for myocarditis. If it is caused by a specific treatable organism, then it is treated with appropriate antibiotics
and anti-toxins. Rest, therapy for heart failure and anti-arrhythmic
drugs are required also. Steroid therapy may also be indicated.

Prognosis
This depends on the aetiology of the myocarditis. Some patients will
die with heart failure or cardiac arrhythmias.

THE CARDIOMYOPATHIES

Cardiomyopathy is a disorder of heart muscle of unknown cause or
association. There are three clinical presentations:

Congestive cardiomyopathy
Hypertrophic (obstructive) cardiomyopathy
Restrictive cardiomyopathy

Cardiomyopathy may be primary or secondary. Examples of secondary
cardiomyopathy include:

Haemochromatosis (a metabolic disease characterized by excessive

deposition of iron in the myocardium and other tissues)
Sarcoidosis
Amyloidosis
Muscular dystrophy

CONGESTIVE CARDIOMYOPATHY

This is the commonest form of cardiomyopathy. The patient often presents with heart failure of unknown aetiology.

Pathology
The heart is grossly dilated and the muscle is pale and soft, but there is no appreciable hypertrophy. There is also extensive damage to the myofibrils.

Haemodynamics
There is decreased contraction of the left ventricle resulting in slow and inaequate systolic emptying. The left ventricle dilates and the pressure rises in the left atrium. Consequently, heart failure and pulmonary hypertension occur.

Clinical features
Dyspnoea. The patient usually presents with dyspnoea and progressively more severe heart failure develops. Increasingly cardiomegaly may precede the symptoms.

Pulses. There is usually tachycardia, atrial fibrillation and ventricular ectopic beats.

Auscultation. Gallop rhythm is common. There may be the pansystolic murmurs of mitral or tricuspid incompetence.

Investigations
ECG. This may show sinus tachycardia, atrial fibrillation or ventricular ectopic beats. There may be non-specific ST and T wave changes. Sometimes left bundle branch block may be present.

Chest X-ray. This confirms the general cardiac enlargement.

Echocardiogram. This shows a poorly contracting and dilated left ventricle. It is useful in assessing cardiomegaly.

Treatment

The main aim is to treat the heart failure. Diuretics are given and digitalis is of use mainly in atrial fibrillation. If severe heart failure persists, oral vasodilators may be of use. Ventricular arrhythmias will probably require specific therapy. If the cardiac output is low, anticoagulants are given to prevent systemic and pulmonary embolism.

Prognosis

The treatment is palliative rather than curative and, generally, cardiomyopathy has a poor prognosis. Cardiac transplantation is not available in most centres, but it is the only definitive treatment.

HYPERTROPHIC CARDIOMYOPATHY

In this form of cardiomyopathy there is marked hypertrophy of the ventricles without any recognized cause. Patients may present with or without outflow tract obstruction. This whole group is often termed Hypertrophic Obstructive Cardiomyopathy (HOCM), or the term in the USA, Idiopathic Hypertrophic Subaortic Stenosis (IHSS) is used.

Pathology

The hypertrophy is usually generalized and may cause obstruction to outflow of the left ventricle. To a lesser degree, there is also obstruction to outflow of the right ventricle. The muscle fibres are abnormally short and thick. The hypertrophy is often most prominent in the ventricular septum.

Haemodynamics

Obstruction by the hypertrophied muscle results in the development of a systolic pressure gradient in the outflow tract of the affected ventricle. This occurs in mid-systole as full contraction develops.

Clinical features.

Dyspnoea. This is due to a high left atrial pressure resulting from the stiff left ventricle.

Angina pectoris. The angina on effort is due to myocardial ischaemia which is caused by the diastolic coronary flow being impeded by abnormal myocardial relaxation. It must be appreciated that the myocardium is hypertrophied out of proportion to the coronary blood supply

Syncope. This is due to a fall in cardiac output.

Palpitations. These may be due to episodic cardiac arrhythmias (ventricular and supraventricular).

Pulses. The pulse is quick-rising due to the rapid ejection of blood by the hypertrophied ventricle during early systole. The venous pulse may show a large 'a' wave, due to forceful atrial contraction against the non-compliant hypertrophied ventricle.

Palpation. Sometimes the cardiac impulse has a double thrust.

Auscultation. A third heart sound is sometimes heard. A fourth heart sound is usual but not always audible. A late systolic murmur is maximal at the left sternal edge and apex.

Investigations
ECG. Often shows evidence of left ventricular hypertrophy. Sometimes there is left bundle branch block.

Echocardiogram. This is usually diagnostic of HOCM. The septum is markedly thick. The mitral valve moves abnormally in that it moves anteriorly during systole. There is also mid-systolic closure of the aortic valve. These latter two are features of the obstructive HOCM.

Chest X-ray. This may show left ventricular hypertrophy.

Cardiac catheterization and angiography. Cardiac catheterization will demonstrate a systolic pressure difference between the body and the outflow tract of the left ventricle if an obstruction is present. Angiography demonstrates a small left ventricular cavity with narrowing of the outflow tract. Sometimes mitral regurgitation is demonstrated.

Treatment
Beta-adrenergic blocking drugs are the main form of treatment for the obstruction and the angina. Diuretics are given only for heart failure. Prophylactic anti-arrhythmic agents and DC cardioversion may be required for dealing with the atrial fibrillation and to deal with any serious arrhythmias. Anticoagulants are required as systemic emboli are a hazard. Surgical treatment is generally reserved for those patients who

do not respond to medical treatment. Surgery usually takes the form of septal resection, and if there is severe mitral valve involvement, mitral valve replacement is indicated. (*Goodwin 1970*)

Prognosis
This is difficult to predict. Patients may survive many years, although the onset of atrial fibrillation is usually a bad sign.

RESTRICTIVE CARDIOMYOPATHY

This is the rarest form of cardiomyopathy. It may easily be misdiagnosed as constrictive pericarditis.

Pathology
Restrictive cardiomyopathy involves an infiltration of the myocardium and endocardium with fibroelastic tissue, similar to that in amyloidosis. The exact pathology is ill-defined.

Haemodynamics
The hypertrophied ventricle is rigid, so it does not distend well in diastole or contract completely in systole. The venous pressure is therefore high and the cardiac output low as in constrictive pericarditis.

Clinical features
The clinical features are usually identical to those of constrictive pericarditis. The distinguishing features may be the lack of evidence of pericardial calcification and the evidence of cardiac enlargement.

Treatment
Treatment of the heart failure is required, as is treatment of any identifiable primary cause. Surgical resection of the fibrous tissue may be considered.

Prognosis
Short term results of surgical intervention are encouraging.

ENDOCARDIUM

The endocardium is the inner layer of the heart. It also forms the heart valves.

The main endocardial disease is inflammation of the endocardium of the heart valves.

ENDOCARDITIS

Endocarditis is an acute or subacute inflammation of the endothelial heart muscle and heart valves.

Acute bacterial endocarditis

This has become rare, except after cardiac surgery and in 'main-lining' drug addicts. Prior to the introduction of antibiotics these patients often died within six weeks.

Subacute bacterial endocarditis

This is the usual form. Although these patients often survived longer than six weeks prior to the introduction of antibiotics, the infections were generally fatal in due course.

BACTERIAL ENDOCARDITIS

This is a relatively rare condition which has a high mortality. This is largely caused by delays in diagnosis.

Aetiology

Bacterial endocarditis may occur in any patient with a cardiac abnormality who has a bacteraemia.

Pathology

Bacteria and fibrin aggregate to form vegetations on the affected valve or cardiac defect. Infected emboli may occur in the systemic circulation if the vegetations are on the mitral or aortic valves. This embolization is frequent and is responsible for many of the clinical features of the disease. Large emboli may cause infarcts in the kidneys, brain, myocardium or lungs. Microemboli affect nearly all parts of the body and are often responsible for skin lesions and a glomerulonephritis. Pulmonary emboli develop when the right side of the heart is involved, as in ventricular septal defect and persistent ductus arteriosus.

Most causes of subacute bacterial endocarditis (SBE) are by organisms of relatively low virulence. The common precipitants of SBE are:

1. Dental procedures: *Streptococcus viridans* is the usual organism here.
2. Genito-urinary and rectal procedures: *Streptococcus faecalis* is the usual organism here.
3. Infected bedsores.
4. Cardiac surgery: *Staphylococcus albus* is a common organism here.

Clinical features

The clinical features in the early stages of the disease are generally unimpressive and may be often overlooked. Short courses of antibiotics may temporarily suppress the infection and make diagnosis more difficult.

Fever. This is often a low-grade fever, associated with cachexia.

Anaemia. The patient is pale as a result of normochromic anaemia. There may be generalized café-au-lait pigmentation of the skin.

Finger clubbing. This develops quickly, but may not be obvious early in the illness.

Diffuse vascular changes. These include glomerular lesions producing red cells in the urine and late renal failure, splinter haemorrhages in the nail beds and generalized cerebral disturbances which may lead to a confusional state.

Emboli. These arise from vegetations on the infected valves. They can vary considerably in size. They may appear in any part of the circulation and present as a cerebral vascular accident or arterial occlusion in the limbs. Recurrent pulmonary emboli are common. Minor emboli in the skin cause painful nodules in the finger pulps. Osler's nodes are larger subcutaneous emboli. Emboli may also be seen in the conjunctivae and in the retina.

Pulses. There is usually a tachycardia and often slight elevation of the venous pressure.

Auscultation. The murmurs appropriate to the underlying valve disease are found. The appearance of a new aortic diastolic or mitral systolic murmur is an indication of infection of the valve, though this may be difficult to assess.

It must be emphasized that this 'typical' picture is no longer common, and the disease is well advanced if all these features are present. A diagnosis should be possible much earlier on the basis of the following:

Fever
Emboli
Changing cardiac murmurs

In a patient with known heart disease these features should always be fully investigated.

Investigations

Blood culture. In many cases a positive blood culture is needed to establish the diagnosis. Six sets of cultures should be taken over a period of hours before antibiotics are given. The blood should be incubated aerobically and anaerobically.

ESR. Elevation of erythrocyte sedimentation rate (ESR) and anti-streptolysin titre (AST) are common, though not specific to SBE.

Echocardiogram. This may help to evaluate the extent of damage to the valve.

Since none of these investigations are specific for bacterial endocarditis, an accurate medical (and dental) history is crucial for diagnosis.

Treatment

This consists largely of antibiotic treatment which is started once the responsible organism has been identified. However, this may have to be initiated before the blood culture result is known. The drug of choice is penicillin because it can be given in high concentrations without toxic effects. However, a combination of antibiotics are often required.

Surgical treatment in the form of aortic or mitral valve replacement may be urgently needed if severe valvular incompetence develops. Surgical treatment is usually successful, provided that effective antibiotic therapy has been started.

Patients with prosthetic valve replacements are at particular risk from endocarditis. If the patient fails to respond to medical treatment, removal of the infected valve and tissues and replacement with a new prosthesis may be successful. (*Weinstein and Rubin 1973*)

Prophylaxis

In susceptible individuals endocarditis can be prevented by an effective level of antibiotic in the blood at the time of the procedure which might lead to a bacteraemia. This applies particularly to those cardiac patients undergoing dental extractions.

Prognosis

Recovery from the disease was rare before the advent of antibiotic therapy. However, antibiotics have significantly reduced the mortality. Death may ensue as a result of heart failure, emboli or renal failure. Even if the endocarditis is cured, damage to the valves may be so serious as to cause intractable heart failure.

REFERENCES

Goodwin, J.F. (1970) Congestive hypertrophic cardiomyopathies. *Lancet, i*, 731.

Hirschmann, J.V. (1978) Pericardial constriction. *Am. Heart J., 96*, 110.

Weinstein, L. & Rubin, R.H. (1973) Infective endocarditis. *Prog. cardiovasc. Dis., 16*, 275.

12
Cardiac Drugs

INTRODUCTION

Common cardiac drugs are discussed where relevant in each section
under the heading of treatment. A more detailed account of each group
of drugs is given in the following pages. This is followed by a section
on cardiac drugs in current use. However, it is by no means complete.

It is important to note that drug therapy is a complex subject and
that new drugs are being introduced on to the market at a rapid rate.

Dosages, where mentioned, are approximations only. The nurse is
strongly advised to read the drug manufacturers data sheet, for a much
more detailed account.

PATIENT COMPLIANCE IN DRUG TREATMENT

In order to achieve maximum patient compliance in taking drugs the
following advice may help the nurse.

Patient education
Over half of the patients who leave hospital have been found to have
a poor or erroneous understanding of their illness and its treatment.
Giving the patient information and taking the time to ensure that this
is properly understood is humane and helpful to the patient. However,

a consistent relationship between this knowledge and good compliance has not been demonstrated.

Reducing the number of tablets to be taken. As would be expected, compliance falls as the number of tablets increases.

Reducing the frequency of tablets to be taken. Again, common sense indicates that this should help compliance.

Clear labelling of containers. Clear instructions (verbal and written) given carefully and rehearsed by the patient may improve compliance. Possibly allowing patients to administer their own drugs while in hospital might be of help.

Other points. The nurse should make the patient aware of any side effects that may occur, and to report these and other problems to his doctor.

CATECHOLAMINES AND SYMPATHOMIMETIC DRUGS

Catecholamines are normally found in sympathetic nerve endings in the heart as well as in arterioles and venules. The principal catecholamine in the heart is noradrenaline (norepinephrine). The heart is capable of functioning normally in the absence of endogenous catecholamines, and in heart failure these stores are depleted. However, sympathetic nerve stimulation is an important supporting mechanism for the heart in the presence of stress.

Catecholamines and other sympathomimetic drugs act upon the circulation by stimulating adrenergic receptors. Adrenergic receptors are classified into two groups, alpha (a) and (β), based on the effects of sympathomimetic amines on a variety of tissue. A further subdivision has been made into β_1 receptors (mainly in the heart) and β_2 receptors (in the peripheral vessels, bronchi and also, possibly, the heart). Beta-adrenergic blocking drugs are *antagonists* of synthetic *agonists* such as isoprenaline and noradrenaline at beta-adrenoceptors.

Stimulation of a-adrenergic receptors results in vasoconstriction, leading to a pressor response. Stimulation of β_1 adrenergic receptors (which are mainly in the heart) results in stimulation of cardiac contractility, automaticity, conduction velocity, and irritability.

SYMPATHOMIMETIC AGENTS

Noradrenaline

Its main action is to stimulate α-adrenergic receptors, thereby producing peripheral vasoconstriction. It also stimulates myocardial β_1-receptors, thereby producing a positive chronotropic and inotropic effect. It is now rarely used as an inotropic agent.

Metaraminol

This is a pressor agent with similar actions to noradrenaline. This, too, is rarely used nowadays.

Isoprenaline

This is a β-adrenergic stimulant. It is effective in stimulating cardiac pacemakers, and therefore may be of benefit in bradycardia or A-V block.

Dopamine

This is the metabolic precursor of noradrenaline, and it also releases noradrenaline from the heart. It has renal and mesenteric vasodilator effects mediated via dopaminergic receptors. It has a half-life of about 2 minutes, and so it is given by IV infusion. Its main uses are in refractory heart failure and in cardiogenic shock or acute myocardial infarction. The most common adverse reaction is tachycardia, which may produce angina.

Dobutamine

This is a synthetic analogue of dopamine. It acts on β_1-adrenergic receptors so as to cause a stronger inotropic rather than chronotropic effect. Unlike dopamine, it does not stimulate the heart indirectly by releasing noradrenaline from nerve endings, nor does it activate dopaminergic receptors. It has a half-life of about 2 minutes, and so it is given by IV infusion. In severe low-output heart failure, it is superior to dopamine.

CARDIOSELECTIVE BETA-BLOCKERS

These drugs inhibit β_1-receptors but exert little influence on the bronchial and vascular β_2-receptors (when used in low doses). This has the advantage that they are safer in patients with obstructive airways disease and make them more suitable for use in hypertension because their use does not block the vasodilator β_2-receptors.

Practolol, metoprolol and atenolol are the only drugs that are truly cardioselective. However, practolol is not available orally on account of its toxicity.

DIGITALIS AND ALLIED CARDIAC GLYCOSIDES

Digitalis and certain other cardiac glycosides have in common a powerful action on the myocardium that is unrivalled in value for the treatment of heart failure.

PHARMACOKINETICS

Some glycosides, including ouabain, are poorly absorbed orally and, therefore, are effective only when administered parenterally. The IV route is preferable to the IM, since absorption with the latter is erratic. When they are administered orally, absorption is nearly complete within 2 hours.

Digoxin

This has a half-life of 1.6 days, and 85% is excreted in the urine. After oral administration, the concentration of digoxin in plasma reaches a peak in 2 - 3 hours, the maximal effect occurring in 4 - 6 hours. If a loading dose of digoxin is not given, up to one week can elapse before steady-state plasma concentrations are obtained.

Digitoxin

This has a half-life of approximately 6 days, and only 15% is excreted in the urine. Because of its long half-life, steady-state plasma concentrations are obtained slowly and recovery from toxicity is protracted. After oral administration, its onset of action is 3 - 6 hours, the maximal effect being apparent in 6 - 12 hours.

Ouabain

This has a half-life of 21 hours. It is very rapid acting, exhibiting an onset of action 5 - 10 minutes and a peak effect 60 minutes after IV injection. It is poorly absorbed from the gastrointestinal tract, and therefore it is not suitable for oral use.

TABLE 5: Dosage and time of effect of digoxin and digitoxin

	Digoxin	Digitoxin
Average digitalizing dose:		
Oral	1.0 - 2.5 mg	0.8 - 1.2 mg
I.V.	0.5 - 2.0 mg	0.8 - 1.2 mg
Average daily maintenance dose:		
Oral	0.125 - 0.75 mg	0.05 - 0.2 mg
I.V.	0.25 mg	0.10 mg
Onset of action:		
Oral	1.5 - 6 hour	3 - 6 hour
I.V.	5 - 30 min.	30 - 120 min.
Maximal effect:		
Oral	4 - 6 hour	6 - 12 hour
I.V.	1.5 - 3 hour	4 - 8 hour

Mechanism of action

The cardiac actions of all digitalis glycosides are the same. They augment contractility and irritability and slow heart rate and A-V conduction. In addition, they potentiate vagal influences on the heart.

The most important effect on cardiac muscle is its increased effect on contractility (positive inotropic effect). The glycosides cause an increased rhythmicity and also prolong the functional refractory period of the A-V node, through a direct action, as well as an enhanced vagal effect. Digitalis also shortens the refractory period of atrial and ventricular muscle. It also exerts a negative chronotropic action, which in part is a vagal effect and in part due to a direct action on the sinus node.

Indications

1. The most important is for heart failure. By stimulating the contractile function of the heart, digitalis improves ventricular emptying.

2. In patients in whom ventricular contractility is impaired secondary to chronic IHD or other forms of heart disease.

3. In preventing or abolishing recurrent episodes of paroxysmal atrial tachycardia. It is also of use in slowing the rapid ventricular rate of patients with atrial fibrillation and flutter.

DIGITALIS INTOXICATION

One would think that the commonest cause of digitalis intoxication would be the ingestion of too large a maintenance dose. However, it is not. The commonest cause is depletion of potassium, which often occurs as a result of diuretic therapy. Other factors which may reduce the tolerance of the patient to digitalis or provoke latent intoxication include: old age, myocardial infarction, hypoxia, DC shock, and magnesium depletion.

Diagnosis of digitalis intoxication

The earliest signs of digitalis toxicity include anorexia, nausea and vomiting. Cardiac arrhythmias that are liable to occur most frequently include ventricular ectopic rhythms, often taking the form of ventricular bigeminy. Variable atrioventricular block may occur, and often accompanies paroxysmal atrial tachycardia. VT and VF may also be induced.

Treatment of digitalis intoxication

Once the diagnosis has been made, treatment is almost always successful. No additional digitalis should be given and diuretics that cause potassium depletion should be withheld. Anti-arrhythmic agents may be required. If potassium is to be given this should be carefully monitored: it is contra-indicated if A-V block is severe. It is important not to administer DC shock therapy in the treatment of digitalis-induced arrhythmias.

DIURETICS

Diuretics are agents that increase the rate of urine formation. A wide variety are now available. Their main use in the context of heart disease is in the treatment of heart failure and hypertension. All the commonly used diuretics act by promoting sodium excretion, with enhanced water excretion as a secondary effect.

Thiazide diuretics

These are widely used because of their effectiveness when administered orally. Their primary action is to decrease sodium reabsorption in the cortical diluting segment of the distal tubule, thus producing an increased excretion of sodium and water. Because of their limited site of action they are only moderately powerful diuretics. Chlorthalidone (which is a diuretic sulphonamide and not a thiazide) is slowly absorbed and therefore has a longer duration of action. Thiazides are usually given orally in the morning and they produce a diuresis through the day.

The chief adverse effect following prolonged administration of these diuretics is potassium depletion. Hypokalaemia can be prevented by giving oral supplements of potassium chloride.

The main indications are:

Heart failure. Thiazides control oedema and dyspnoea, and in many patients, including those in whom oedema is not clinically apparent, they are more effective than digitalis in controlling symptoms.

Hypertension. Thiazides have anti-hypertensive properties although their mode of action is not fully understood. Thiazides may be used alone or in conjunction with other agents such as beta-blockers and vasodilators.

TABLE 6: Common thiazide and related diuretics currently in use in UK

Drug	Usual daily dose range (mg)	Duration of action (hours)
Chlorothiazide	500 - 2000	10
Hydrochlorothiazide	25 - 100	10
Bendrofluazide	2.5 - 10	20
Cyclopenthiazide	0.25 - 1.0	12
Chlorthalidone	50 - 200	48

High-ceiling or loop diuretics

These are extremely powerful diuretics. They prevent reabsorption at multiple sites including the proximal and distal tubules and the ascending limb of the loop of Henle. They induce a peak diuresis far greater than that observed in other agents, and they have a rapid onset of action.

The three loop diuretics are:

Frusemide
Bumetanide
Ethacrynic acid

The main use of these drugs is in the urgent treatment of heart failure.

Supplements of potassium chloride should be given to all patients receiving these drugs.

Potassium-sparing diuretics

These are diuretics which do not cause potassium loss. They are not very powerful and are often combined with other diuretics.

Potassium sparing diuretics include:

Amiloride
Triamterine
Spironolactone

ANTI-ARRHYTHMIC DRUGS

It is important to realise that if the plasma potassium level is kept below 4.5 mmol/litre, this may decrease the incidence of arrhythmias.

TABLE 7: Classification of anti-arrhythmic agents

Class		Drugs
I.	Membrane-stabilizing agents	(a) Quinidine and quinidine-like agents (including procainamide & disopyramide)
		(b) Lignocaine and lignocaine-like agents (including phenytoin, mexiletine, and tocainide)
		(c) Others: propranolol
II.	Beta-blocking agents	Propranolol and all other beta-blockers
III.	Agents widening action-potential duration	Amiodarone
IV.	Calcium-antagonist agents	Verapamil (anti-arrhythmic effect not yet shown for other calcium-antagonists)

It has recently been postulated that increased free fatty acids (FFA) may play a role in the genesis of arrhythmias during acute myocardial infarction, and that glucose can reverse some of the electrophysiological abnormalities of elevated FFA.

Classification of anti-arrhythmic agents

Four classes of anti-arrhythmic agents have been described by *Vaughan Williams (1980)*, and these are outlined in Table 7. Anion antagonists may be a fifth class of anti-arrhythmic action *Millar and Vaughan Williams 1981)*.

Beta-adrenergic blocking drugs

These drugs are used especially for supraventricular tachycardia provoked by emotion and exercise, and in chronic ventricular arrhythmias when heart failure is absent. The evidence that they prevent sudden death in IHD is inconclusive.

The drugs most commonly used are propranolol (Inderal) and practolol (Eraldin), though the latter is no longer available orally.

Lignocaine (Lidocaine, Xylocard)

This is the standard parenteral agent for suppression of ventricular arrhythmias (ventricular ectopic beats and ventricular tachycardia) associated with acute myocardial infarction. When given orally, only 30% of the drug is available. In addition, oral administration is associated with greater CNS effects.

Lignocaine has a half-life of 120 minutes. The conventional regimen is an IV bonus followed by a reducing infusion rate.

The efficacy of lignocaine in preventing VF is the subject of some debate.

Mexiletine (Mexitil)

This is similar in structure to lignocaine but is not rapidly metabolised by the liver. It is sometimes described as an 'oral lignocaine' and may be effective in lignocaine-resistant arrhythmias. Its major use is in the chronic oral prophylaxis of ventricular arrhythmias, especially after acute myocardial infarction.

Mexiletine has a half-life of 16 – 18 hours. It is well absorbed orally, but absorption is delayed after infarction. The usual regimen is an IV bolus followed by a reducing infusion rate until oral therapy is established.

Phenytoin (Epanutin, Dilantin)

This is an effective anti-arrhythmic agent, although it is mainly used as an anti-convulsant. Its main use is in the treatment of digitalis-induced ventricular arrhythmias, because it increases A-V nodal conduction but decreases ventricular excitability.

Procainamide (Pronestyl)

This is effective in many arrhythmias but is not now popular because of its side effects (it may induce a systemic lupus erythematosus syndrome after long-term use). Although largely supplanted by lignocaine, it may suppress ventricular arrhythmias when other agents have failed.

The value of sustained-release procainamide is not yet fully realized.

Bretylium tosylate

This is an effective drug against ventricular fibrillation refractory to lignocaine and multiple DC shocks. In other ventricular arrhythmias, the drug takes a long time to act.

Quinidine

Despite the advent of new anti-arrhythmic agents, quinidine still has a place. It depresses excitability, conduction velocity and contractility of the heart. It also lowers peripheral resistance. Its main use now is as a prophylactic agent in preventing arrhythmias (supraventricular and ventricular). It can be given orally, IM or IV, but the latter route is extremely dangerous. Sustained-release quinidine (Kinidin Durules) is now the preferred form.

Quinidine has a half-life of 5 – 7 hours. It is rapidly and almost completely absorbed. Phenobarbitone and phenytoin reduce plasma quinidine levels and efficacy. Quinidine may raise plasma digoxin concentrations 2-3 fold.

Disopyramide (Rythmodan, Norpace)

This is very similar to quinidine, although some of the electrophysiological properties resemble those of lignocaine. It has a half-life of 6 – 8 hours. It can be used in the treatment of supraventricular and ventricular arrhythmias, although recently the drug has come under some harsh criticism because of its side effects, especially in relation to inducing heart failure. However, the drug is effective in the prophylaxis of arrhythmias after acute myocardial infarction and in reducing the recurrence of arrhythmias after cardioversion.

Verapamil (Cordilox)

This is a calcium-ion antagonist which was first used as an anti-anginal agent and is now widely prescribed for cardiac arrhythmias. It is used in the acute therapy of supraventricular arrhythmias, but does not seem useful in ventricular arrhythmias. It is used mainly in tachyarrhythmias associated with Wolff-Parkinson-White syndrome. (*Anonymous 1981*)

Verapamil must not be used if the patient is already receiving a beta-blocking drug, because the interaction of these two may produce severe bradycardia, and asystole.

Amiodarone (Cordarone X)

This is a new anti-arrhythmic agent which has been proved to be of value in the treatment of cardiac arrhythmias resistant to other therapy. It has a prolonged action, and can be given once daily, on a low dosage. Experience with IV amiodarone shows that it is rapidly effective for supraventricular tachycardias with a maximum effect 10 minutes after injection. It is of use in patients with recurrent VT and VF. (*Chapman and Boyd 1981*)

Tocainide

This is a new drug which is an oral lignocaine analogue. It can also be given IV. The effects of the drug are not yet fully known as it has only been used recently. It has been reported to be effective against potentially dangerous arrhythmias refractory to quinidine, procainamide, and propranolol.

Atropine

Atropine is an anticholinergic agent. It has a half-life of 13 – 38 hours.

Its main clinical use in cardiology is in the treatment of sinus bradycardia, junctional rhythm and transient second-degree A-V block.

NITRATES

Nitrates have been used successfully for over a century in the treatment of angina. Their mechanism of action has already been covered (Chapter 7). They may be divided into short and long acting.

SHORT-ACTING NITRATES

Glyceryl trinitrate

This is the most important agent used in the therapy of angina. It can be given in the sublingual form or intravenously. With sublingual GTN clinical effects begin within two minutes and last for us to an hour. The half-life is 7 minutes. GTN paste applied to the chest provides prolonged release, and can be wiped off in the event of an adverse reaction.

It is important that the nurse appreciates that sublingual GTN is sometimes ineffective, probably because the patient has not been given the proper information.

LONG-ACTING NITRATES

Isosorbide dinitrate
Long-acting nitrates are a controversial issue. However, for the patient requiring protection for several hours, they do have advantages.

CALCIUM ANTAGONISTS

Calcium-ion antagonists are a new class of drugs that are proving very successful in cardiology. There are four in clinical use in the UK. These are:

Verapamil
Nifedipine
Prenylamine
Perhexiline

Inhibition of calcium uptake by myocardial cells depresses contractility, thus reducing oxygen requirements and decreasing the response to sympathetic stimulation. The heart rate usually falls, which also reduces oxygen demand. These drugs are also vasodilators, particularly nifedipine.

Verapamil was first used as an anti-anginal agent and is now widely used as an anti-arrhythmic agent. Nifedipine was first used as an anti-anginal agent and is now being used for the treatment of hypertension.

VASODILATORS

These drugs have recently regained popularity in the treatment of hypertension and of heart failure.

Nitroprusside
This drug has a direct action on the smooth muscle of arteries and

veins. It has an immediate action, with the half-life being in the order of seconds. It is used mainly for severe low-output left heart failure, but is useful in selected patients with myocardial infarction and left-ventricular failure. It is very effective in hypertensive crises (especially those associated with LVF), and to a lesser extent in the control of dissecting aortic aneurysm. It is also used to reduce afterload in the management of cardiogenic shock and in hypotensive anaesthesia.

The nurse must be aware of certain factors associated with this potent drug. The infusion rate needs careful titration against the patient's blood pressure, using an infusion pump or microdrip regulator. It must not be stopped abruptly. The infusion should be shielded from light. Cyanide may accumulate with prolonged high doses. This can be avoided by monitoring blood thiocyanate levels.

Hydralazine

This is also a direct-acting vasodilator: It has a direct action on the smooth muscle of arteries and has a half-life of 2–4 hours. In hypertension, hydralazine is best combined with a beta-blocker and diuretics. In heart failure, it is best combined with nitrates.

Metabolism of hydralazine occurs by hepatic acetylation. Therefore, it is important to ascertain the patients *acetylation status*. Patients who are fast acetylators have lower steady-state plasms concentrations, less reduction in blood pressure and a reduced incidence of side effects, in comparison to those patients who are slow acetylators.

Prazosin

This is described as an 'oral nitroprusside' because it dilates both peripheral arterial and peripheral venous systems, thus decreasing the blood pressure and increasing the cardiac output. Its action appears to be due to a-blockade. Its major use therefore, is in the treatment of hypertension. It has a half-life of 4 hours, but little is known about its metabolism.

Diazoxide

This is a direct-acting arteriolar vasodilator which is an analogue of the thiazide diuretics. It also causes catecholamine release. It has a long half-life of 20 – 30 hours. It has many severe side effects, including sodium retention, hyperglycaemia and hypersensitivity. Therefore, its main use is in the emergency treatment of severe hypertension.

Minoxidil

This is a new vasodilator which is still undergoing investigation. Its action is the same as diazoxide. It also has severe side effects. Minoxidil is being used for hypertension, but needs to be given in conjunction with beta-blockers and diuretics.

Labetalol

This drug has mixed a- and β-blocking properties, being much less pronounced at a-receptors. Some of its properties are similar to prazosin, with a half-life of $3 - 4$ hours. It has an immediate hypotensive effect, and is used in moderate and severe hypertension, sometimes in combination with a diuretic or methyldopa.

Phentolamine

This is primarily an a-blocking agent, but it may also act to release noradrenaline. Its main use is as an intravenous arteriolar vasodilator in low-output left-ventricular failure.

SOME COMMON CARDIAC DRUGS

This section deals with four main areas of therapy for cardiovascular disease: angina, hypertension, heart failure and cardiac arrhythmias.

ANGINA

Drugs used in the treatment of angina include glyceryl trinitrate, beta-adrenergic blocking drugs, perhexilene, and occasionally verapamil.

HYPERTENSION

Drugs used in the treatment of hypertension include diuretics, beta-adrenergic blocking drugs, vasodilators, and other anti-hypertensives such as methyldopa and labetalol.

HEART FAILURE

Drugs used in the treatment of heart failure include diuretics (often combined with potassium supplements), digoxin and other inotropic agents such as dopamine, and vasodilators.

ARRHYTHMIAS

Drugs used in the treatment of cardiac arrhythmias include digoxin, beta-adrenergic blocking drugs, verapamil, lignocaine and disopyramide.

Acebutolol (Sectral)
Beta adrenergic blocking drug with limited cardioselectivity.

Use: In angina, hypertension and cardiac arrhythmias.

Dose: 100 – 400 mg twice daily orally.

Side effects: Bronchoconstriction, heart failure and cold extremities.

Adrenaline (Epinephrine)
Adrenergic cardiac stimulant.

Use: In cardiac arrest.

Dose: 1 – 5 ml of 1/10 000 sol. IV bolus or intracardiac.

Side effects: Fear, anxiety, headache, sweating, pallor, respiratory difficulty and apnoea, hypertension, pulmonary oedema and cardiac arrhythmias.

Alprenolol (Betacard, Aptin)
Beta adrenergic blocking drug.

Use: In angina, hypertension and cardiac arrhythmias.

Dose: 400 – 800 mg daily orally.

Side effects. Bronchoconstriction, heart failure and cold extremities.

Amiloride Hydrochloride (Midamor)
Potassium sparing diuretic.

Use: In treatment of oedema. Often combined with a thiazide.

Dose: 10 – 20 mg daily orally.

Side effects: Dizziness and weakness.

Aminophylline (Cardophylin)
Respiratory and cardiac stimulant.

Use: In heart failure, pulmonary oedema and Cheyne-Stokes respiration.

Dose: 100 – 300 mg orally. Suppositories of 360 mg. 250 mg in 10 ml water slowly IV.

Side effects: Nausea and vomiting if given orally; vertigo, restlessness, cardiac arrhythmias if given IV.

Atenolol (Tenormin)
Beta adrenergic blocking drug with cardioselectivity.

Use: In angina, hypertension and cardiac arrhythmias.

Dose: 100 – 200 mg orally daily.

Side effects: Bronchoconstriction, heart failure and cold extremities.

Atropine Sulphate
Anticholinergic.

Use: In sinus bradycardia, digitalis toxicity and vaso-vagal attacks.

Dose: 0.6 mg (600 mcg) IV bolus.

Side effects: Dry mouth, pupillary dilatation, urinary retention, dehydration and tachycardia.

Bendrofluazide (Aprinox)
Thiazide diuretic.

Use: In treatment of oedema and in control of hypertension.

Dose: 2.5 – 10 mg orally daily.

Side effects: Potassium depletion, hyperglycaemia, glycosuria and gout.

Bethanidine (Esbatal)
Adrenergic blocking drug.

Use: Treatment or hypertension.

Dose: 10 – 100 mg twice daily orally.

Side effects: Postural hypotension, dizziness, fluid retention and impotence.

Bretylium (Darenthin)
Adrenergic blocking drug.

Use: Ventricular ectopic beats, tachycardia and fibrillation, and other cardiac arrhythmias.

Dose: 100 – 200 mg three times a day orally.

Side effects: Hypotension.

Bumetanide (Burinex)
Potent diuretic

Use: In treatment of oedema and heart failure.

Dose: 1 – 2 mg daily orally.

Side effects: Potassium depletion.

Calcium chloride
Cardiac stimulant.

Use: Cardiac arrest.

Dose: 10 ml of 10% sol. IV bolus or intracardiac.

Side effects: Cardiac arrhythmias, (in digitalized patients), vasodilation, hypotension, bradycardia, syncope.

Clonidine (Catapres)
Antihypertensive.

Use: In treatment of hypertension.

Dose: 0.05 – 0.2 mg three times a day orally.

Side effects: Drowsiness, sedation, headache and dizziness.

Diamorphine (Heroin)
Narcotic analgesic.

Use: In treatment of heart failure and management of myocardial infarction.

Dose: 5 mg IM.

Side effects: Vomiting, hypotension, respiratory depression and addiction. Use antiemetic at same time.

Digoxin
Inotropic agent.

Use: In treatment of heart failure, atrial fibrillation and flutter, and in supraventricular tachycardia.

Dose: Digoxin dose schedules vary. In adult: 0.5 mg t.d.s. for 1 day. 0.25 mg q.d.s. for 1 day, 0.25 mg t.d.s. for 1 day, then 0.25 mg daily or b.d. maintenance, orally.

Side effects: Depends on serum potassium levels and kidney function. Common are anorexia, nausea and vomiting, malaise with headaches, visual disturbances, ventricular ectopic beats, coupling of beats and all grades of atrioventricular block.

Disopyramide (Norpace, Rythmodan)
Anti-arrhythmic.

Use: Ventricular ectopic beats, tachycardia and fibrillation and other cardiac arrhythmias.

Dose: 100 – 200 mg three times daily orally.

Side effects: Dry mouth, blurred vision, bradycardia, and cardiac standstill.

Dopamine (Intropin)
Adrenergic; inotropic agent.

Use: In treatment of shock.

Dose: IV infusion 5 mcg/kg/min up to 20 – 50 mcg/kg/min.

Side effects: Palpitation, vasoconstriction, hypotension, angina, tachycardia and ectopic beats.

Ethacrynic Acid (Edecrin)
Potent diuretic.

Use: In treatment of oedema and heart failure.

Dose: 50 mg three times a day orally.

Side effects: Potassium depletion, hyperglycaemia, glycosuria and gout.

Frusemide (Lasix)
Potent diuretic.

Use: In treatment of oedema.

Dose: 40 – 80 mg or more daily orally. 20 – 40 mg IV.

Side effects: Potassium depletion, hyperglycaemia, glycosuria and gout.

Note: Reserved for patients who are resistant to thiazides, or are in acute heart failure.

Glyceryl Trinitrate
Vasodilator.

Use: Relief of angina.

Dose: 0.5 mg sublingually.

Side effects: Headache, dizziness and flushing.

Guanethidine (Ismelin)
Adrenergic blocking drug.

Use: Treatment of hypertension.

Dose: 25 – 50 mg daily. Up to 300 mg daily in severe hypertension.

Side effects: Postural hypotension, fluid retention and impotence.

Heparin
Anticoagulant.

Use: Prevention of thrombosis.

Dose: 15 000 units IV 12 hourly.

Side effects: Allergic reactions and, on prolonged use, osteoporosis. Heparin-induced haemorrhage controlled by protamine sulphate.

Hydralazine (Apresoline, Rolazine)
Vasodilator.

Use: Hypertension.

Dose: 25 – 200 mg twice daily orally.

Side effects: Headaches, flushing, SLE syndrome.

Isoprenaline (Isoproterenol)
Cardiac stimulant.

Use: Treatment of cardiac arrest. In a long-acting form is of value in treatment of chronic heart block.

Dose: 0.01 – 0.05 mg IV or intracardiac. 10% sol. at 1 ml/min IV infusion.

Side effects: Apprehension, palpitations, tachycardia and other arrhythmias.

Labetalol (Trandate)
Antihypertensive.

Use: Hypertension.

Dose: 100 – 800 mg three times daily orally.

Side effects: Postural hypotension, bronchospasm, heart failure and lethargy.

Lignocaine (Lidocaine, Xylocaine)
Anti-arrhythmic.

Use: Ventricular ectopic beats, tachycardia and fibrillation.

Dose: 1 mg/kg IV stat., then 1 mg/min infusion.

Side effects: Confusion, convulsion and coma.

Metoprolol (Betaloc, Lopressor)
Beta adrenergic blocking drug with cardioselectivity.

Use: In angina, hypertension and cardiac arrhythmias.

Dose: 50 – 200 mg twice daily orally.

Side effects: Bronchoconstriction, heart failure and cold extremities.

Methyldopa (Aldomet, Dopamet)
Antihypertensive.

Use: Hypertension.

Dose: 250 – 1000 mg three times daily orally.

Side effects: Sedation, depression and impotence.

Mexiletine (Mexitil)
Antiarrhythmic.

Use: Ventricular ectopic beats, tachycardia and fibrillation.

Dose: 100-200 mg IV. 400 mg stat. orally, then 200 mg three times daily.

Side effects: Nausea, dizziness, visual disturbance, hypotension and bradycardia.

Oxprenolol (Trasicor)
Beta adrenergic blocking drug.

Use: Angina, hypertension and cardiac arrhythmias.

Dose: 20 - 80 mg or more three times daily orally.

Side effects: Bronchoconstriction, heart failure and cold extremities.

Perhexilene (Pexid)
Anti-anginal agent.

Use: Treatment of angina.

Dose: 100 - 200 mg twice daily orally.

Side effects: Dizziness, nausea, vomiting, weakness, flushing and skin rashes.

Phenytoin (Epanutin)
Antiarrhythmic.

Use: Ventricular ectopic beats, tachycardia and fibrillation, and other cardiac arrhythmias.

Dose: 100 mg three times daily orally. 100 - 300 mg IV.

Side effects: Ataxia, dysarthria and nystagmus.

Practolol (Eraldin)
Beta adrenergic blocking drug with cardioselectivity.

Use: In cardiac arrhythmias.

Dose: 5 mg slowly IV (Maximum 20 mg). Not now available orally.

Side effects: Bronchoconstriction, heart failure and cold extremities.

Procainamide (Pronestyl)
Anti-arrhythmic.

Use: Ventricular ectopic beats, tachycardia and fibrillation.

Dose: 250 – 500 mg four times daily orally.

Side effects: Hypotension systemic lupus erythematosus (SLE) syndrome.

Propranolol (Inderal)
Beta adrenergic blocking drug.

Use: In angina, hypertension and cardiac arrhythmias.

Dose: 40 – 360 mg three times daily orally.

Side effects: Bradycardia, hypotension, heart failure, bronchoconstriction and depression.

Quinidine (Kinidin Durules)
Anti-arrhythmic.

Use: Ventricular ectopic beats, tachycardia and fibrillation, Also atrial arrhythmias.

Dose: 500 – 1250 mg twice daily orally (slow release).

Side effects: Nausea, cinchonism (tinnitus, dizziness, headache), hypersensitivity, ventricular arrhythmias.

Spironolactone (Aldactone)
Aldosterone antagonist.

Use: Potentiation of diuretics and prevention of potassium depletion.

Dose: 50 – 200 mg daily.

Side effects: Hyperkalaemia, gynaecomastis.

Streptokinase
Fibrinolytic agent.

Use: Thrombotic or embolic disease.

Dose: 100 000 – 500 000 units IV, then 200 000 units for four hours and 100 000 units per hour for up to three days in an infusion.

Side effects: Allergic reactions, haemorrhage.

Verapamil (Cordilox)
Anti-arrhythmic.

Use: Supra-ventricular and other tachycardias.

Dose: 40 – 120 mg three times daily orally.

Side effects: Nausea, hypotension and bradycardia.

REFERENCES

Anonymous (1981) Calcium antagonists and the heart. *Br. med. J.*, *1*, 89.

Chapman, J.R. & Boyd, M.J. (1981) *Intravenous amiodarone in ventricular fibrillation. Br. med. J.*, *1*, 951.

Millar, J.S. & Vaughan Williams, E.M. (1981) Anion antagonism — a fifth class of anti-arrhythmic action? *Lancet*, *i*, 1291.

Vaughan Williams, E.M. (1980) *Anti-arrhythmic action.* London: Academic Press Inc. (London) Ltd.

COMMON CARDIOVASCULAR ABBREVIATIONS

AAT	—	Aspartate aminotransferase
ACG	—	Apexcardiogram
ASD	—	Atrial septal defect
AV	—	Atrioventricular
BCR	—	British corrected ratio
BPM	—	Beats per minute
CAD	—	Coronary artery disease
CCU	—	Coronary care unit
CHD	—	Coronary heart disease
CPK	—	Creatine phosphokinase
CPR	—	Cardiopulmonary resuscitation
CVP	—	Central venous pressure
ECG	—	Electrocardiogram
HDL	—	High density lipoprotein
IABP	—	Intra-aortic balloon pump
ICU	—	Intensive care unit
IHD	—	Ischaemic heart disease
LAD	—	Left anterior descending coronary artery
LAP	—	Left atrial pressure
LCA	—	Left coronary artery
LDH	—	Lactic dehydrogenase
LDL	—	Low density lipoprotein
LVEDP	—	Left ventricular end-diastolic pressure
LVF	—	Left ventricular failure
LVH	—	Left ventricular hypertrophy
MCL	—	Mid-clavicular line
PAP	—	Pulmonary arterial pressure
PCO_2	—	Partial pressure of carbon dioxide
PCG	—	Phonocardiogram
PDA	—	Patent ductus arteriosus
PO_2	—	Partial pressure of oxygen
PWP	—	Pulmonary wedge pressure
RAP	—	Right atrial pressure
RCA	—	Right coronary artery
RHD	—	Rheumatic heart disease
SA	—	Sinoatrial
SBE	—	Subacute bacterial endocarditis
VSD	—	Ventricular septal defect

INDEX